Quality Improvement

Editors

TREASA 'SUSIE' LEMING-LEE
RICHARD WATTERS

NURSING CLINICS
OF NORTH AMERICA

www.nursing.theclinics.com

Consulting Editor
STEPHEN D. KRAU

March 2019 • Volume 54 • Number 1

ELSEVIER

1600 John F. Kennedy Boulevard • Suite 1800 • Philadelphia, Pennsylvania, 19103-2899

http://www.theclinics.com

NURSING CLINICS OF NORTH AMERICA Volume 54, Number 1
March 2019 ISSN 0029-6465, ISBN-13: 978-0-323-65515-6

Editor: Kerry Holland
Developmental Editor: Casey Potter

Nursing Clinics of North America (ISSN 0029-6465) is published quarterly by Elsevier Inc., 360 Park Avenue South, New York, NY 10010-1710. Months of issue are March, June, September, and December. Periodicals postage paid at New York, NY and additional mailing offices. Subscription price per year is, $163.00 (US individuals), $491.00 (US institutions), $275.00 (international individuals), $598.00 (international institutions), $231.00 (Canadian individuals), $598.00 (Canadian institutions), $100.00 (US students), and $135.00 (international students). To receive student/resident rate, orders must be accompanied by name of affiliated institution, date of term, and the signature of program/residency coordinator on institution letterhead. Orders will be billed at individual rate until proof of status is received. Foreign air speed delivery is included in all *Clinics* subscription prices. All prices are subject to change without notice. **POSTMASTER:** Send address changes to *Nursing Clinics*, Elsevier Health Sciences Division, Subscription Customer Service, 3251 Riverport Lane, Maryland Heights, MO 63043. **Customer Service: Telephone: 1-800-654-2452** (U.S. and Canada); **1-314-447-8871 (outside U.S. and Canada). Fax: 1-314-447-8029. E-mail: journalscustomerservice-usa@elsevier.com** (for print support) and **journalsonlinesupport-usa@elsevier.com** (for online support).

Nursing Clinics of North America is covered in *EMBASE/Excerpta Medica, MEDLINE/PubMed (Index Medicus), Social Sciences Citation Index, Current Contents, ASCA, Cumulative Index to Nursing, RNdex Top 100,* and Allied Health Literature and International Nursing Index (INI).

Contributors

CONSULTING EDITOR

STEPHEN D. KRAU, PhD, RN, CNE
Associate Professor (Ret), Vanderbilt University School of Nursing, Nashville, Tennessee

EDITORS

TREASA 'SUSIE' LEMING-LEE, DNP, MSN, RN
Assistant Professor of Nursing, Director of Organizational Performance Improvement, Vanderbilt University School of Nursing, Nashville, Tennessee

RICHARD WATTERS, PhD, RN
Associate Professor of Nursing, Vanderbilt University School of Nursing, Nashville, Tennessee

AUTHORS

AMY J. COSTANZO, PhD, RN-BC
Nursing Administration, University of Cincinnati Medical Center, Cincinnati, Ohio

TERRI DAVIS CRUTCHER, DNP, MSN, RN
Assistant Professor, Interim Academic Director, Nursing and Health Care Leadership Assistant Dean, Clinical and Community Partnerships, Vanderbilt University School of Nursing, Nashville, Tennessee

KRISTIN A. CUMMINS, DNP, RN
Associate Chief Nursing Officer, Executive Director of Pediatric and Maternal Quality and Safety, Quality and Safety Department, Riley Hospital for Children at Indiana University Health, Indianapolis, Indiana; DNP Student, Vanderbilt University, Nashville, Tennessee

GORDON LEE GILLESPIE, PhD, DNP, RN, CEN, CNE, CPEN, PHCNS-BC, FAEN, FAAN
Professor and Deputy Director for Graduate Occupational Health Nursing Program, College of Nursing, University of Cincinnati, Cincinnati, Ohio

JANE GOETZ, MSN, RN, NEA-BC
Nursing Administration, University of Cincinnati Medical Center, Cincinnati, Ohio

DENISE K. GORMLEY, PhD, RN
University of Cincinnati College of Nursing, Cincinnati, Ohio

ADELAIDE N. HARRIS, DNP, MSN, MEd, RN
Assistant Professor, Clinical Nursing, University of Cincinnati College of Nursing, Academic Health Center, Cincinnati, Ohio

KIMBERLY HIGGINBOTHAM, DNP, APRN, CPNP, PMHS
Associate Professor, Assistant Dean, Director of Graduate Nursing Programs, Cedarville University, School of Nursing, Cedarville, Ohio

JESSICA HILL-CLARK, MBA, MA
University of Cincinnati College of Nursing, Cincinnati, Ohio

KRISTYN C. HUFFMAN, DNP, RN, AGACNP-BC
University of Arizona College of Nursing, Tucson, Arizona

JAHMEEL ISRAEL, MS
University of Cincinnati College of Nursing, Cincinnati, Ohio

SHARON M. KARP, PhD, MSN, RN, CPNP-PC
Assistant Professor of Nursing, Vanderbilt University School of Nursing, Nashville, Tennessee

TREASA 'SUSIE' LEMING-LEE, DNP, MSN, RN
Assistant Professor of Nursing, Director of Organizational Performance Improvement, Vanderbilt University School of Nursing, Nashville, Tennessee

JOANNE PHILLIPS, DNP, RN, CNS, CPPS
Director of Clinical Practice, Virtua Health System, Marlton, New Jersey

BONNIE PILON, PhD, RN-BC, NEA, FAAN
Professor Emerita, Vanderbilt University School of Nursing, Vanderbilt University, Nashville, Tennessee

SHEA POLANCICH, PhD, RN
Assistant Dean, Clinical Innovation for Quality Improvement, UAB Nursing Partnership, UAB School of Nursing and UAB Hospital, The University of Alabama at Birmingham, Birmingham, Alabama

ROSEMARY C. POLOMANO, PhD, RN, FAAN
Associate Dean for Practice, Professor of Pain Practice, University of Pennsylvania School of Nursing, Professor of Anesthesiology and Critical Care (Secondary), University of Pennsylvania Perelman School of Medicine, Philadelphia, Pennsylvania

TRACY PRITCHARD, PhD
University of Cincinnati College of Nursing, Cincinnati, Ohio

JENSINE A. RUSSELL, DNP, RN
Nurse Manager, Inpatient Medicine, Vanderbilt University Medical Center, Nashville, Tennessee

KATHERINE STAUBACH, MSN, MEd, RN, CPPS
Nursing Administration, University of Cincinnati Medical Center, Cincinnati, Ohio

RICHARD WATTERS, PhD, RN
Associate Professor of Nursing, Vanderbilt University School of Nursing, Nashville, Tennessee

LYDIA J. YEAGER, DNP, MSN, RN, CPNP-PC
School Based Health Program Manager, Ryan Health, New York, New York

Contents

Using knowledge gained from the disciplines of nursing, medicine, health care management, and medical and health services research, the quality improvement movement attempts to mobilize people within the health care system to work together in a systematic way using evidence based strategies and tactics to improve the care they provide. In this valuable work, discipline-specific knowledge is combined with experiential learning and discovery to make improvements. Quality improvement provides a knowledge-based framework and methods for the change agent to work toward a more predictable, effective, efficient, reliable, equitable, patient-centered care health care system.

The purpose of this quality improvement study was to describe the process for workplace aggression (WPA) reporting and the potential failures for this process in a pediatric emergency department. Interviews were conducted with 10 interdisciplinary employees. Findings yielded 7 tasks following WPA: contact security, contact police, contact clinical manager, notify emergency department director, call safety hotline, complete electronic safety form, and complete paper safety form. Focusing actions to prevent failure modes and causes for (1) notification of the emergency department director and (2) completion of an electronic safety form can garner the greatest improvement in overall risk for WPA reporting.

Fast tracks are widely used in emergency departments to increase patient throughput as annual visits continue to rise in the United States. A modified triage process known as QuickLook, which omits patients' past medical history, is used in some hospitals to further increase throughput. This article discusses the effects of QuickLook on patient placement, reviews

recommended nurses lead this change through innovative models of patient-centered care and IPCP participation. One strategy to improve patient experience is rounding. This project presents a nurse-led interprofessional bedside rounding model to improve communication and collaboration between providers and with patients on a complex inpatient unit. Outcomes were analyzed using Hospital Consumer Assessment of Healthcare Providers and Systems (HCAHPS) scores to examine patient experience. Postimplementation results demonstrate an increase in HCAHPS patient experience scores for this patient population above hospital and national average.

Reducing Pressure Injuries in the Pediatric Intensive Care Unit

Kristin A. Cummins, Richard Watters, and Treasa 'Susie' Leming-Lee

This quality improvement project used the Model for Improvement including the Plan-Do-Study-Act cycle of change framework to educate pediatric intensive care unit (PICU) nurses on risk factors for pediatric pressure injuries and prevention strategies, improve turning compliance for PICU patients, and implement an electronic trigger to order nutrition consultations on all patients with a Braden Q score less than 16. The quality improvement project decreased preventable patient harm to PICU patients by decreasing the pressure injury incidence rate from 8% to 3% in the 6-week time period.

Screening for Social Determinants of Health at Well-Child Appointments: A Quality Improvement Project

Kimberly Higginbotham, Terri Davis Crutcher, and Sharon M. Karp

Children living in poverty are vulnerable to the adverse effects associated with unmet basic needs, such as food and housing. Poverty threatens the overall growth and development of children placing them at risk for poor cognitive, behavioral, and psychological outcomes. Addressing social determinants of health in the pediatric primary care setting is within the role of the pediatric primary care provider. The Model for Improvement guided this quality improvement project in the implementation of food and housing insecurity screening during well-child appointments in a rural health clinic.

Diabetes Self-management Education Provision by an Interprofessional Collaborative Practice Team: A Quality Improvement Project

Adelaide N. Harris

Please note that citations/references numbers are not included in abstracts; please modify if needed: Diabetes is a major health problem and requires patients with diabetes to gain knowledge to manage their care effectively. The shift in diabetes care is to focus teaching on self-management to engage and empower patients with diabetes to live the best quality of life. Health care providers may not always be aware of diabetes self-management education available to patients. The American Association of Diabetes Educators has identified 7 essential self-care behaviors known as AADE7. The focus of this quality improvement project is to increase the provision and documentation of diabetes self-management education at a health center in Cincinnati, Ohio.

This project applied a quality improvement design to assess perceived barriers to pediatric overweight and obesity guideline implementation in school-based health centers. An electronic survey was administered to nurse practitioners and licensed practical nurses working in school-based health centers in New York. The most commonly cited primary care–based barriers were lack of patient compliance, family lifestyle, and the poor dietary practices and sedentary behaviors common in America. The most commonly cited school-based barriers were that children have little control over the groceries purchased and foods cooked at home and the lack of parent presence during appointments.

NURSING CLINICS OF NORTH AMERICA

SERIES OF RELATED INTEREST

Critical Care Nursing
Available at: https://www.ccnursing.theclinics.com/

THE CLINICS ARE AVAILABLE ONLINE!
Access your subscription at:
www.theclinics.com

Foreword

Quality Improvement: Evolution or Revolution?

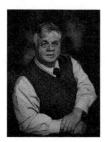

Stephen D. Krau, PhD, RN, CNE
Consulting Editor

Is Quality Improvement (QI) the result of evolution or the result of evolution? This question has been the focus of discussion in nursing and health care for decades. In retrospect, it seems to have been both, but in hindsight, the current phenomenon has been the result of evolution. Quality management in the United States can be traced to the 1920s and to the initiatives of Edward Deming, Walter A. Shehart, and Joseph Juran, who laid the groundwork for health care initiatives. [1] Not many decades ago, what we now consider Quality Improvement was called "Quality Assurance" or "Quality Management." Quality assurance in the health care setting often consisted of a few people, who were not necessarily nurses, who compiled and analyzed data related to "incident reports," now often referred to as "occurrence screenings," which consisted of mostly medication errors, aberrant and negative happenings, patient lengths of stay, and patient satisfaction indicators. Often these satisfaction indicators were unsolicited feedback as the result of patients who experienced some component of a hospital stay.

The shift in terms from quality "assurance" to quality "improvement" indicates a change in thought and purpose. "Assurance" indicates that there is a binding commitment to do, or give, or refrain from something. It is a pledge, in this case, of quality. It is not transitional, nor does it indicate movement. "Improvement" is an occasion when something gets better or when you make it better.[2] The term indicates movement in the sense of progression, advancement, or development. Change is fundamental to improvement, just as it is to QI. The evolution of QI has been long, challenging, and active. It has involved many people, organizations, regulatory agencies, and legislation.

It is very inviting to treat improvement initiatives as though they are stable and undaunted by the environment in which they occur. To do this would simplify the matter and make these initiatives so much simpler. Health care systems, and life in general, are not that simple. Experienced improvers know that the actions introduced to a health care system to change things for the better involve a dynamic and complex process of "flex and morph."[3]

Nurs Clin N Am 54 (2019) xi–xii
https://doi.org/10.1016/j.cnur.2018.12.002
0029-6465/19/© 2018 Published by Elsevier Inc.

The importance of nurse involvement in QI is well supported and is a very logical fit. When considering the improvement of care for patients, it is the nurse who provides continuous care and who provides ongoing assessments, interacts with the families of patients as well as the patient, provides treatment and medications, and educates patients and families. As part of the evolutionary process of QI, there have been many groups and agencies that have developed and supported quality indicators to measure outcomes of care in the health care environment, systems to address the economic aspects of care delivery, and to "minimize overall human suffering during illness."[1] Many of these groups and organizations are discussed in this issue of *Nursing Clinics of North America*.

Draper and colleagues[4] explain how nurses play a pivotal role in helping hospitals meet QI guidelines, define initiatives for QI, and thereby enable hospitals and other health care settings to effectively use the expert role of the nurse in quality improvement. Challenges to nurses in the role of improvers are immense. Some of these challenges include the adequacy of nursing staff when resources are scarce, engaging nurses at all levels in QI initiatives, increasing QI initiatives, and the lack of nurse preparation in traditional nursing education for the nurse's role in quality efforts.

In 2008, "The Essentials of Baccalaureate Education for Professional Nursing"[5] was revised and directed that students participate in the retrieval, appraisal, and synthesis of evidence to improve patient outcomes. This requirement also requires collaboration in these processes with other members of the health care team. This is a clear indication of the evolutionary process of QI not only in the health care facilities themselves but also in the academic institutions that educate nurses to become improvers of quality patient outcomes. The guest editors for this issue of *Nursing Clinics of North America*, Drs Leming-Lee and Watters, have assembled an impressive collection of articles on QI, the aim of which is to provide evidence, examples, and data for the improvement of patient outcomes.

Stephen D. Krau, PhD, RN, CNE
Vanderbilt University School of Nursing
6809 Highland Park Drive
Nashville, TN 37205, USA

E-mail address:
steve.krau@vanderbilt.edu

REFERENCES

1. Owens LD, Koch RW. Understanding quality patient care and the role of the practicing nurse. Nurs Clin North Am 2015;50(1):33–43.
2. Cambridge Dictionary. Available at: https://dictionary.cambridge.org/dictionary/english/improvement. Accessed November 28, 2018.
3. Marshall M, de Silva D, Cruickshank L, et al. What we know about designing an effective improvement intervention (but too often fail to put into practice). London: University College London; 2016. Available at: http:dx.doi.org/10.1136/bmjqs-2016-006245. Accessed November 30, 2018.
4. Draper BM, Selanders LC, Beck DM, et al. The role of nurses in hospital quality improvement, vol. 3. Washington, DC: Center for Studying Healthcare System Change. Available at: www.hschange.com/CONTENT/972/972.pdf. Accessed November 30, 2018.
5. American Association of Colleges of Nursing. The essentials of baccalaureate education for professional nursing practice 2008. Available at: www.aacn.nche.edu/education resources/baccessentials08.pdf. Accessed November 28, 2018.

Preface

Quality Improvement

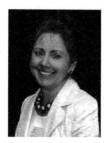
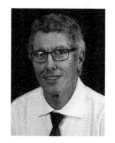

Treasa 'Susie' Leming-Lee, DNP, MSN, RN   Richard Watters, PhD, RN

Editors

REFLECTION

Before we introduce you to the March 2019 issue of the *Nursing Clinics of North America* devoted to quality improvement in the delivery of health care, we would like you to think about quality improvement and its impact on the health care industry and health services organizations during the last 1 to 3 years. How do we translate "best practice" to our health care organizations?

Although we have made significant progress to improve health care and value, reform policy, increase access and equitability, and reduce costs of care, we continue to be challenged by high costs, poor health care outcomes, and our ability to translate evidence-based strategies and tactics into everyday practice. Health spending is a significant part of our economy, which accounted for 17.2% of the US gross domestic product (GDP) in 2017.[1] The GDP is a measure of all goods and services produced by a nation in a given year; it is the nation's income, in the form of goods and services. In light of the GDP, the rate of health care consumption in the United States is much higher than other high-income countries, greater than the second (Switzerland, 12.3%) and third (France, 11.5%) highest spenders. The lowest spenders are Turkey (4.2%) and Mexico (5.4%), less than 6% of their respective GDPs on health care.[1]

It is expected that health spending per capita in 2017 will be greater than USD 10,000 in the United States. Per capita spending in Switzerland (USD 8009) and Luxembourg (USD 7049) is much less than in the United States.[1] The expenditures continue to increase every year.

Nurs Clin N Am 54 (2019) xiii–xv
https://doi.org/10.1016/j.cnur.2018.12.001
0029-6465/19/© 2018 Published by Elsevier Inc.

nursing.theclinics.com

An examination of health care system performance across 11 countries in 2017 revealed that the United States ranked last overall. They also ranked last in access, equitability, and health care outcomes. The United States ranked fifth in care process.[2] The analyses also indicated that there were noticeable variations among the domains of performance. In essence, no country ranked first across every domain; all countries have opportunity to improve.

The current infrastructure for quality improvement in health care is the result of a long history of efforts to improve the quality of care and health outcomes. It involved the recognition of the role of quality in health care, prioritization of quality improvement, and the development and implementation of systems and processes to monitor, track, and reward quality improvement in health care. As we are all too familiar, there have been numerous attempts to address the challenges associated with quality improvement.

By the end of the twentieth century, there were a number of reports that revealed "strong evidence of widespread quality deficiencies and highlighted a need for substantial change to ensure high-quality care for all patients."[3] The Institute of Medicine's (IOM) *To Err is Human: Building a Safer Health System*[4] and *Crossing the Quality Chasm: A New Health System for the 21st Century*[5] are seminal reports that continue to highlight the challenges and opportunities to improve the quality of health care in the United States. The IOM (2000) revealed that 100,000 deaths in the United States annually were due to preventable errors. Subsequent to this report, the IOM (2001) recommended the following aims to improve quality of care in the twenty-first century: safe, effective, patient-centered, timely, efficient, and equitable.

Moving forward, the IOM's report on *The Future of Nursing*[6] made a number of recommendations to support the contributions of nurses to improve the health of the US population. The report described the study context as evolving health care challenges; quality, access, and value as primary concerns in health care reform; and principles of change. Recommendation #1, Expand opportunities for nurses to lead and diffuse collaborative improvement efforts, and Recommendation #7, prepare and enable nurses to lead change to advance health, clearly support nurses' efforts and future efforts to improve the quality of health care delivery.

Although significant progress has been made in translating evidence-based practice and quality improvement, discussions with nurse leaders, advanced practice nurses, registered nurses, and other health care providers reveal one of the greatest challenges is to change practice to reflect *best practice* based on evidence-based practice. Although the evidence supports "best practice," why is it so difficult to implement *best practice* in our organizations based on evidence-based practice? In other words, the evidence supports "best practice," but we are challenged to implement the change. The challenge often resides in the context of your health care organizations within which the planned change is to occur.

In selecting the quality improvement projects for this issue of *Nursing Clinics of North America*, we chose authors and quality improvements from across the country, including various heath care organizations. The purpose of this collection of quality improvement projects is to share examples of quality improvement projects and different processes that can be used to implement change in the respective health care organizations. The authors and we hope the collection of quality improvement projects will engage your interest and stimulate thoughts and ideas about how to make change to improve health care quality and value, translating *best practice* within the context of your respective health care organizations in a cost-effective manner.

Treasa 'Susie' Leming-Lee, DNP, MSN, RN
Vanderbilt University School of Nursing
461 21st Avenue South
216 Godchaux Hall
Nashville, TN 37240, USA

Richard Watters, PhD, RN
Vanderbilt University School of Nursing
461 21st Avenue South
220 Godchaux Hall
Nashville, TN 37240, USA

E-mail addresses:
susie.leming-lee@vanderbilt.edu (T.'S.' Leming-Lee)
Richard.watters@vanderbilt.edu (R. Watters)

REFERENCES

1. Organisation for Economic Co-operation and Development (OECD). Health statistics 2018. Available at: http://www.oecd.org/els/health-systems/health-data.htm. Accessed July 23, 2018.
2. Schneider EC, Sarnak DO, Squires D, et al. Mirror, mirror 2017: international comparison reflects flaws and opportunities for better US health care. The Commonwealth Fund; 2017. Available at: https://interactives.commonwealthfund.org/2017/july/mirror-mirror/?_ga=2.213791124.1230998792.1532121939-394285837.1532121939#chapter5. Accessed July 23, 2018.
3. Joshi MS, Ransom ER, Nash DB, et al. The healthcare quality book: vision, strategies, and tools. 3rd edition. Chicago (IL): Health Administration Press; 2014.
4. Institute of Medicine (IOM). To err is human: building a safer health system. Washington, DC: National Academy Press; 2000.
5. Institute of Medicine (IOM). Crossing the quality chasm: a new health system for the 21st century. Washington, DC: National Academy Press; 2010.
6. Institute of Medicine (IOM). The future of nursing: leading change, advancing health. Washington, DC: The National Academies Press; 2011.

Translation of Evidence-Based Practice

Quality Improvement and Patient Safety

Treasa 'Susie' Leming-Lee, DNP, MSN, RN[a],*,
Richard Watters, PhD, RN[b]

KEYWORDS

- Evidence-based practice • Quality improvement • Patient safety

KEY POINTS

- Healthcare providers must reframe the healthcare experience to discover new solutions and possibilities for better healthcare delivery, they must become the change agents.
- Improvement comes from the application of knowledge, the more complete the appropriate knowledge, the better the improvement will be when this knowledge is applied to making change.
- The science of improvement is a multidisciplinary disciple drawing on clinical science, systems theory, statistics, psychology, and other fields.
- A translation gap exists between what is known about evidence-based practice and implementation of best practice by health care providers.
- Evidence based practice (EBP) frameworks and models have the potential to increase the use of evidence to guide the care process.

Powerful forces of change are at work within the American health care system. The public debate concerning health care financing and access to insurance coverage is intensifying. But, below the surface of the media and policy debate about cost and access, a quieter but perhaps more significant process of change is under way: the transformation of health care management and delivery—indeed, health professional work itself—through health care quality improvement. The innovative, interdisciplinary quality improvement movement has begun to significantly upgrade delivery of health care in the United States. Taking its cue from reform approaches in other industries, and driven especially by studies indicating a shockingly widespread incidence of medical errors and a striking lack of consistency in the standard of care patients receive in different facilities and from different practitioners, the quality improvement movement has arrived in health care.[1]

a Vanderbilt University School of Nursing, 461 21st Avenue South, 216 Godchaux Hall, Nashville, TN 37240, USA; b Vanderbilt University School of Nursing, 461 21st Avenue South, 220 Godchaux Hall, Nashville, TN 37240, USA
* Corresponding author.
E-mail address: susie.leming-lee@vanderbilt.edu

Nurs Clin N Am 54 (2019) 1–20
https://doi.org/10.1016/j.cnur.2018.10.006
0029-6465/19/© 2018 Elsevier Inc. All rights reserved.

Using knowledge gained from the disciplines of nursing, medicine, health care management, and medical and health services research, the quality improvement movement attempts to mobilize people within the health care system to work together in a systematic way using evidence-based strategies and tactics to improve the care they provide. In this valuable work, discipline-specific knowledge is combined with experiential learning and discovery to make improvements.[1]

Because of this powerful transformation, health care providers must reframe their vision of how to deliver patient care through a different lens. They must be able to find simplicity and order amid a chaotic health care system.[2] Health care providers must also be artists who are versatile and flexible, as well as analysts, who can reframe the health care experience to discover new solutions and possibilities for better health care delivery, they must become the change agents.[2] As the change agent, there is a need for knowledge and methods to meet this new vision for delivering patient care. Quality improvement provides a knowledge-based framework and methods for the change agent to work toward a more predictable, effective, efficient, reliable, equitable, patient-centered care health care system.

WHAT IS QUALITY IMPROVEMENT?

To define quality improvement, there is a need to first define quality. "Quality is not a physical attribute of a service or product—it does not exist until there is an interaction between the product or service and the person making the judgment. Quality is a perception that is based on an individual's value system."[3(p17)] Quality is meeting or exceeding customer requirements.[3] Understanding the definition of quality gives meaning to the work of quality improvement. Perla and colleagues[4] describe quality improvement as a trial and error approach for making change grounded in testing and learning cycles. "Improvement comes from the application of knowledge-of medicine, engineering, teaching, driving a truck, or simply the way some activity is currently done. Generally, the more complete the appropriate knowledge, the better the improvement will be when this knowledge is applied to making change."[5(p3)]

Health Care Quality Improvement

The Institute of Medicine's report, *Crossing the Quality Chasm: A New Health System for the 21st Century*, which raised serious doubts about the quality of health care in the United States, defines health care quality improvement as the degree to which health services for individuals and populations increase the likelihood of desired health outcomes and are consistent with current professional knowledge.[1] The Institute of Medicine report[6(p6)] recommended the following 6 aims or dimensions of health care quality:

(a) safe, avoiding injuries to patients from the care that is intended to help them; (b) effective, providing services based on scientific knowledge to all who could benefit, and refraining from providing services to those not likely to benefit; (c) patient-centered, providing care that is respectful of and responsive to individual patient preferences, needs, and values, and ensuring that patient values guide all clinical decisions; (d) timely, reducing waits and sometimes harmful delays for both those who receive and those who give care; (e) efficient, avoiding waste, including waste of equipment, ideas, and energy; (f) equitable, providing care that does not vary in quality because of personal characteristics such as gender, ethnicity, geographic location, and socioeconomic status.

Health care quality improvement can also be defined as "a process for producing excellent outcomes using evidenced-based medicine and best clinical skills to meet the needs and expectations of consumers."[7(p34)] Within this definition are several of the core quality improvement activities, such as: "(1) to seek an understanding of the sources of systematic as well as unwanted and unnecessary variation, (2) implementation of cost-effective and efficient, waste reducing strategies to remove unwanted variation, and (3) to produce organization-wide knowledge on structured approaches to change processes and improve outcomes."[7(p34)]

"Quality improvement involves these core activities in a way that uniquely defines its discipline. Understanding variation and raising outcomes to a higher level requires thinking from a systems point of view."[7] Improvement that is effective and efficient requires data-driven methods and ongoing evaluation. Continuous learning occurs through shared knowledge within an organization that embraces management through team work, leadership in strategic planning, alignment of support services, suppliers and distributors, and reflection on results.[7]

Variation
Understanding the concept of variation is essential to improvement work. What is variation? It is "any quantifiable difference between individual measurements; such difference can be classified as being due to common cause (random) or special causes (assignable)."[8(p341)] Interaction among process variables, including materials, methods, procedures, people, equipment, information, measurement, and environment, produces sources of variation. The primary purpose of understanding variation is to enable predictions (Speroff, personal communication, 2001) which is a component of the scientific method. Shewhart's theory of chance cause variation differentiates between common and special causes of variation in data.[9] Common causes are "those causes that are inherent in a system (process or product) over time, affect everyone working in the system, and affect all outcomes of the system."[10(p30)] Special causes are "those causes that are not always part of a system (process or product) or do not affect everyone, but arise because of specific circumstances."[10(p30)]

Stable and unstable processes
A process or system that only has common causes affecting the measurement of interest is called a stable process. A stable process is one in which the cause system for the measure of interest remains essentially constant over time. A stable process, in the state of statistical control, implies only that the variation in outcomes to expect in the future is predictable within limits, not that it has desirable or undesirable performance.[9,10]

A process with outcomes affected by common and special causes is called an unstable process for the measure of interest, with the magnitude of the variation from one time period to the next being unpredictable. As special causes are identified and appropriately acted on, the process becomes stable. The "theory of variation provides a basis for action to improve a system. A stable system requires a fundamental change to affect its future performance (because it is stable), while an unstable system requires local action depending on the special cause. In addition to providing the basic concepts of the theory of variation, Shewhart also introduced the control chart method to determine whether variation in a process is due to common or special causes."[10(p30)] This control chart, a time series graph, is a simple and effective way to define the voice of the process that signals that something has changed in the process (special cause) or is it just noise in the process (common variation).[11] Variation is key to understanding how to improve a process or system,[12] and it is vital that all quality improvement providers understand the concept.

IMPROVEMENT SCIENCE IN HEALTH CARE

What is "improvement science"? What is the intellectual foundation of improvement science? What does it look like in real-world applications? What, if anything, might we, as nurses, learn from the techniques and tools of improvement science?[13]

The concept of "improvement science" is frequently used interchangeably with "science of improvement," "continuous improvement," "system improvement," and "scientific quality improvement," to name but a few.[14] The term science of improvement surfaced in Langley and colleagues's[5] publication titled, *The Improvement Guide: A Practical Approach to Enhancing Organizational Performance.*

Lemire and colleagues[13(p25)] consider Deming's system of profound knowledge as the "intellectual foundation for improvement science, the pillars on which improvement science is grounded." The system of profound knowledge is, "a map of theory by which to understand the organizations we work in."[9(p92)] The term profound denotes insight into a knowledge that offers how to make changes that result in an improvement in a variety of settings such as health care, education, the automobile industry or the nuclear power industry. The interdependence of the system's 4 domains: (a) appreciation for a system—understanding how the system works, (b) knowledge about variation—what is the variation trying to tell us about a process and the people who work in it, is the process in a stable or unstable state, (c) theory of knowledge—a concern for how people's view of what is meaningful knowledge is impacts their learning and decision making, and (d) psychology—understanding how the interpersonal and social structures impact performance of a process or system, are defined by Deming as the system of profound knowledge.[5] Deming saw the system of profound knowledge as the route to transformation of a system. This approach is called the science of improvement.[15]

Based on Deming's system of profound knowledge, Langley and colleagues[5] identified 2 critical ideas to help define the science of improvement: (1) improvement arises from developing, testing, and implementing changes and (2) subject matter expert is the lead in developing changes and creating the conditions for testing.[4] Lemire and colleagues[13(p25)] define improvement science as:

A data-driven change process that aims to systematically design, test, implement, and scale change toward systematic improvement, as informed and defined by the experience and knowledge of subject matter experts.

Quality improvement is the trial and error approach for making change. "Improvement comes from the application of knowledge-of medicine, engineering, teaching, driving a truck, or simply the way some activity is currently done. Generally, the more complete the appropriate knowledge, the better the improvement will be when this knowledge is applied to making change."[5(p3)] "The science of improvement is an applied science that stresses innovation, rapid-cycle testing in the field and spread of outcomes to generate learning about what changes, in which contexts, produce improvements."[15(p2)] Characteristics of the science of improvement include a combination of expert subject knowledge along with improvement methods, such as a statistical approach to reducing variation, and the improvement science strategy, and tools, such as control charts used to stabilize the variation.[15] The science of improvement is also a multidisciplinary disciple drawing on clinical science, systems theory, statistics, psychology, and other fields.[15]

According to Langley and colleagues,[16(p75)] "science refers to a system of acquiring knowledge of the physical world. This system must be based on observable phenomena and capable of being tested through the scientific method for it validity. Acquiring knowledge is essential for improvement activities, whether it is a simple problem to solve, a work process to improve, a design or redesign of a product or service, or improvement to a complex system." The most obvious question is: What type of knowledge will allow us to develop, test, and implement changes that result in improvement? Subject matter knowledge acquired through formal and informal learning and reinforced with experiences is the most obvious and appropriate answer to this question. Subject matter knowledge is vital for developing changes that will result in improvement and is basic to the activities we do in life.[5] "Effective changes must be informed by the experiences, knowledge, and intuitions of subject matter experts who are closest to the problems, but to be most effective, these insights must be framed scientifically and tested."[4(p172)] Just as clinical practitioners combine knowledge of biomedical data with individual patient's needs and preferences, continuous improvement practitioners integrate knowledge of generalizable scientific evidence with unique clinical practice environment.

The clinical improvement equation facilitates such reflective practice to ensure sustained and meaningful change grounded in the full spectrum of knowledge systems.[17] Engagement in improvement work brings these separate knowledge systems to life and compels the improvement practitioners to unify these systems for the purpose of optimizing patient care.[17]

To help us understand the operationalization–application of improvement science, Perla and colleagues[4] identified seven propositions that provide the improvement scientist with a clear, concise understanding of how to conduct improvement work. The seven propositions are grounded in the history and philosophy of science, coming together to inform the nature of the science of improvement.[4] The seven propositions of the science of improvement are[4(p173)]:

1. The science of improvement is grounded in testing and learning cycles.
2. The philosophic foundation of the science of improvement is conceptualistic pragmatism.
3. The science of improvement embraces a combination of psychology and logic (eg, a weak form of psychologism).
4. The science of improvement considers the contexts of justification and discovery.
5. The science of improvement requires the use of operational definitions.
6. The science of improvement employs Shewhart's Theory of cause systems.
7. Systems theory directly informs the science of improvement.

Table 1 briefly describes the seven propositions and what it means to applying improvement methods.

Langley and colleagues[5] and Perla and colleagues[4] provide a strong argument for the science of improvement based on its philosophic and theoretical foundations. Perla and colleagues[4] state that, if improvement efforts and projects in health care are to be characterized under the canon of science, there is a need for health care professionals engaged in quality improvement work to ensure there is a standard set of core principles, as standard lexicon, and most important an understanding of the evolution of the science of improvement.

Improvement initiatives, the vehicle for change, are designed to contribute to micro-system learnings rather than to generalizable knowledge[18] as are clinical research studies which challenge the reliability and validity of such initiatives. Walsh states[19(p57)]:

[Q]uality improvement initiatives are complex social interventions, for which high levels of variance in context, content and application are often inherent and

Table 1
Seven propositions of the science of improvement

Seven Propositions (Perla et al,[4] 2013)	Brief Summary Description of Proposition	What Proposition Means to Applying Improvement Methods
1. The science of improvement is grounded in testing and learning cycles.	• Leads to the justification of the PDSA cycles of improvement as an approach that is aligned with the scientific method.	• The PDSA approach requires that a predication (hypothesis) is described, that the data are collected to test the prediction, the analysis of the data are used to determine whether the prediction is correct or not, and the results generate learning and forms the basis for the next improvement cycle test.
2. The philosophic foundation of the science of improvement is conceptualistic pragmatism.	• Leads to the importance of using prior and existing knowledge to form theories, develop changes, and make predictions as to what will happen when these changes are applied. This proposition also supports the use of the Shewhart control charts as to tools to measure existing system performance and to guide future prediction of the system performance.	• Conceptualistic pragmatism states that everyone's observations are informed by their past experience (conceptualistic). In turn, these experiences are used to predict a range of possible futures what can be acted on (pragmatic). Inferring from these underlines the importance of forming theories from existing knowledge and then predicting what will happen as these theories are applied in the form of change concepts. Studying data over time through Shewhart's control chart methodology and theory of variation is central to improvement methods and reflects Lewis' pragmatism.
3. The science of improvement embraces a combination of psychology and logic (eg, a weak form of "psychologism").	• Provides the basis for multidisciplinary collaboration addressing problems from different perspectives, which is one psychology attribute of Deming's system of profound knowledge. This proposition underlines why it is important to use social sciences approaches in the improvement methods and activities.	• Psychologism is a view that acknowledges that both psychology and formal ways of knowing such as analytical philosophy, logic, and mathematics are essential to understanding human behavior and decision making. This idea was once rejected by Western philosophers, but is now considered a critical component to the science of improvement focusing on understanding the multiple dimensions of thought and action.

(continued on next page)

Table 1 (continued)		
Seven Propositions (Perla et al,[4] 2013)	**Brief Summary Description of Proposition**	**What Proposition Means to Applying Improvement Methods**
4. The science of improvement considers the contexts of justification and discovery.	• Reinforces the notion that improvement efforts always involve a component of discovery and creativity in problem solving. These activities must be balanced by some form of justification, such as using data to know if the tests of change worked, how well the change worked, and what will be the next steps in the improvement process.	• The context of justification answers the questions, "what do we know" and "how do we know" while the context of discovery is focused on the processes of discovery and innovation, which are fluid and dynamic. Both justification and discovery are core quality improvement concepts and there is a focus on rapidly testing ideas to determine if and to what degree the concepts work.
5. The science of improvement requires the use of an operational definition.	• Emphasizes the need for improvers to develop consistent, clear definitions of the terms they use. The improvers must also ensure that others involved in improvement understand those definitions to have a shared understanding.	• Operational definitions provide a method for developing a shared meaning and understanding of concepts, ideas, goals/aim, and measures. Without operational definitions, the meaning and intent of words and actions are only known by the individuals who use them. Collective action and effective communication require that all involved in the improvement initiative be on the same page; operational definitions are designed to minimize confusion and move those involved toward a shared understanding.
6. The science of improvement uses Shewhart's Theory of cause systems.	• Stresses understanding variation using improvement tools, such as Shewhart's control charts. These tools allow us to understand whether a process is stable or in control and to distinguish between process special and common cause variation.	• Shewhart's control chart method is more than a statistical tool, it is a theory of variation and the voice of the process. The focus of the control chart is on learning whether a process is stable, in control, and can be used to determine whether the implemented changes made to a system result in improvement. The idea of a "chance-cause" system indicates that a process will behave within certain normal (random) limits based on the system, this is the voice of the process. If there is a failure to recognize this chance-cause system this leads to the risk of tampering with a stable system, the effect of which can often be increased variation and poorer performance.

(continued on next page)

Table 1 (continued)		
Seven Propositions (Perla et al,[4] 2013)	Brief Summary Description of Proposition	What Proposition Means to Applying Improvement Methods
7. Systems theory directly informs the science of improvement.	• Provides the basis for Deming's System of Profound Knowledge component, Appreciation for a System. This component focuses on system thinking, which means viewing the organization as dynamic, adapting to the customer's needs, and is composed of interdependent people, departments, processes, equipment, products, and facilities, all working toward a common purpose or aim.	• The thought processes, the language, and the systems theory methods of understanding is critical to leading improvement. Systems thinking linked with the pragmatism of proposition 2 and Shewhart's theory of variation in proposition 3 leads to Deming's concept of analytical studies. System's thinking provides a focus on how the components relate to each other as a whole to create a system. Systems thinking is not a natural act, so it is essential to become comfortable with system's thinking to keep the focus on how the parts of a system care connected, rather than the performance of the parts of the system.

Abbreviation: PDSA, plan, do, study, act.
Data from Perla RJ, Provost LP, Parry GJ. Seven propositions of the science of improvement: exploring foundations. Qual Manag Health Care 2013;22(3):170–86.

desired characteristics of the initiative. For example, the responses of different healthcare organizations to a continuous quality improvement programme, or system for adverse event reporting and investigation, will be quite different – and the programme or system will be rightly tailored or modified to make it work better in the individual organizational setting. Attempts to 'standardize' or control such interventions to make them fit an experimental paradigm completely misses the point - that their multiple outcomes are a complex co-product of context, content and application variables.

Health care clinicians who are asked to either lead and/or participate in improvement initiatives often ask for evidence that the initiative will work and without existing evidence will resist improvement initiatives. For the science of improvement methodology to be adopted in health care, there needs to be a clear understanding of the similarities and differences between the science of quality improvement and the science for clinical research.

QUALITY IMPROVEMENT MODELS

Why do we need a model to design, develop, implement, and evaluate quality improvement initiatives? If there is no model, it is difficult to assess causal linkages between structure and care processes and/or the impact of these linkages on outcomes.[21] A model provides for a systematic approach[20] to improvement not only guiding the design of an improvement project, but also the data collection, analysis, and interpretation of the results.[21] Using a model ensures that you are not missing any of the critical improvement project steps. However, no one model meets the need of all situations in need of improvement.[22]

There are many quality improvement models used to guide improvement projects. We want to focus on the most commonly used frameworks based on Deming's work, the Model for Improvement (MFI), which was created by Associates for Process Improvement. This simple, effective, and reliable framework is used to bring about successful process or system change.[15] The MFI benefits both the novice and expert quality improvement practitioners because[23(para4)]:

- It is a simple approach that anyone can apply
- It reduces risk by starting small test of change
- It can be used to help plan, develop, and implement change
- There is sufficient evidence that the model is highly effective.

The MFI has 2 equal parts: 3 fundamental questions and the plan–do–study–act cycle to test changes in the practice setting. The 3 fundamental questions are:

- What are we trying to accomplish? To answer this question, we need to develop an aim statement for the project that is specific, measurable, attainable, realistic, and time limited.
- How will we know that a change is an improvement? To answer this question, we need to develop measures that will assess the progress made toward the aim.
- What change can we make that will result in improvement? To answer this question, we need to generate change ideas that will lead to accomplishing the aim.[15]

Although the MFI is the most commonly used improvement framework, we also want to introduce and briefly describe 4 other models, the Toyota Production System Model, the Lean Model, DMAIC (Six Sigma), DMADV (a version of Six Sigma), and FADE (**Table 2**).[24–28] In reviewing each of the models, you may notice that planning, implementation, analysis, and review are common elements in each of them.

TRANSLATING EVIDENCE: THEORIES AND FRAMEWORKS

Translating research evidence into action contributes to better quality health care and health outcomes. Unfortunately, a gap still exists between what is known about evidence-based practice (EBP) and implementation of best practice by health care providers, including registered nurses.[29] Kanter and associates[30] estimate that it takes about 17 years for the implementation of EBPs into clinical practice. Schuster and co-workers[31] conducted a review of published studies on quality of care received. The findings indicated that 70% of people received recommended acute care, 60% received recommended chronic care, and 50% received recommended preventive care.

Although there is a wide range of strategies for implementing best practice, barriers still exist in translating evidence. The Agency for Health Care Policy and Research[32] implemented the Translating Research into Practice to evaluate strategies for translating research findings into practice. The aim of the Translating Research into Practice-II program was to identify sustainable and reproducible strategies and methods to speed up the impact of health services research on direct patient care and improve outcomes.[33] Farquhar and associates[34] studied the projects and found that the most common Translating Research into Practice intervention for translation was education and the most common framework was adult learning theory or organizational theory.

In light of the complex and dynamic nature of the health care environment, health care providers are challenged to respond to this rapidly changing landscape. The concept of change is integral to quality improvement and patient safety. The design,

Table 2
Quality improvement models/methodologies

QI Models:	MFI (Model for Improvement), a PDSA Model Can Be Used as a Stand-Alone Model	Toyota Production System (Lean) Model	DMAIC (Six Sigma)	DMADV (Six Sigma)	FADE
Description	A 2-part problem solving model. *Part 1,* the "thinking part" focuses on 3 questions to set the aim, establish measures, and select changes. This is the strategy component of the model. *Part 2,* the "doing part," using the Plan-Do-Study-Act cycles 4-step cycle for problem solving to test changes on a small scale. This is the tactic component of the model. *Plan:* Hypothesize what will happen; develop action plan solutions. *Do:* Implement possible solutions. *Study:* Evaluate the results to build new knowledge. *Act:* Adopt results, abandon results, or run through the cycle again, possibly under different conditions, different materials, different people or different rules. Langley et al,[16] 2009	A model that is used to remove waste (8 wastes: [1] defects, [2] over-production, [3] waiting, [4] confusion, [5] motion/ travel, [6] excess inventory, [7] overprocessing, and [8] human creativity) from the process or system; defines value by customer (ie, patient) requirements. Maps how the value flows (process) to the customer and ensuring non-valued-added steps are removed from the process leading to a more effective and time efficient process. Langley et al,[16] 2009	A model that uses the Six Sigma measurement based strategy model for process improvement and problem solving. DMAIC is designed to examine existing processes. HRSA,[25] 2016	A model that uses the Six Sigma measurement based strategy model for process using DMADV, which is like the DMAIC but instead of using control for process improvement to examine existing processes, the terms design and verify are used to develop new processes. HRSA,[25] 2016	FADE, a model used for process improvement and problem solving; it that has 4 components: (1) focus (identification of improvement opportunity), (2) analyze (information gathering), (3) develop (create implementation plan and probable solution), and (4) execute (execute plan and monitor results). Duke University,[26] 2016
Aim/goal	Reduce variation	Reduce waste	Reduce variation	Reduce variation	Reduce variation

Application guides				
1. What are we trying to accomplish (aim)?	Identify value; Set target to understand value stream; Develop countermeasures	Define	Define	Focus
2. How will we know a change is an improvement (measures)?	Try countermeasures	Measure	Measure	Analyze
3. What changes can we make that will result in improvement (changes)?	Monitor both processes and results; Eliminate waste	Analyze	Analyze	Develop
Plan	Standardize successful processes; Establish flow	Improve	Design	Execute
Do				
Study	Enable pull; Identify gaps for next steps; Pursue new knowledge	Control	Verify	Evaluate
Act	Moen & Norman,[27] 2006	Liker & Franz,[28] 2011		

Data from Refs.[23–26]

implementation and evaluation of quality improvement projects involves change. Health care leaders require the knowledge, skills, and attitudes to not only improve the quality of patient care, but sustain and spread improvements. The 5 Million Lives Campaign refers to sustainability as "locking in the progress that hospitals have made already and continually building upon it."[35(p3)] Spread is "actively disseminating best practice and knowledge about every intervention and implementing each intervention in every available care setting."[35] Leadership plays an integral role in the assessment of an organization's readiness to sustain and spread the improvement.

EBP frameworks and models have been used to guide the implementation of EBP. These frameworks and models have the potential to increase our use of evidence to guide care, to guide the process. Our health care organizations should adopt the EBP models that further the organization's mission and vision, strategic management plan of the organization that best fits their context of care, aligns with improvement goals, addresses priority problems, and guides a systematic and evaluative approach to collaborative practice change. The IOWA model of research-based practice to promote quality of care and The Johns Hopkins Nursing EBP model and guidelines are described as examples of EBP frameworks and models. These 2 models are often used to guide the design, implementation and evaluation of an EBP change.

The Iowa Model of Evidence-Based Practice to Promote Quality Care

The Iowa Model of Evidence-Based Practice to Promote Quality Care[36] is a useful guide for nurses and other health care providers, as well as multidisciplinary teams to facilitate the integration of EBP for change improvement. The Iowa model is a multiphase change process based on the problem solving steps in the scientific process.[37] Starting points, decision points, and feedback loops are integral to evaluating change. McEwen and Wills[38] report the Iowa model is one of the best researched EBP models.

The Iowa model uses triggers, that is, clinical problems focused or knowledge focused from within or outside the organization to initiate the EBP change process. As the team progresses through the algorithm, they answer questions at decision points to ultimately promote quality care based on the strength and value of the evidence. If the change is appropriate for adoption, the team implements the change. If not, the team continues to evaluate new knowledge and quality of care.

The Johns Hopkins Nursing Evidence-Based Practice Model and Guidelines

The Johns Hopkins Nursing Evidence-Based Practice model was developed by a collaborative team of nurse leaders from the Johns Hopkins Hospital and the Johns Hopkins University School of Nursing. The purpose was to accelerate the transfer of research to practice and to increase nurse autonomy, leadership, and engagement with interdisciplinary colleagues.[39] The model consists of a conceptual model, a process, and tools to guide nurses through the steps of the process.

The Johns Hopkins Nursing Evidence-Based Practice model is a problem-solving approach that uses, as its essential ingredient, the best available evidence for clinical decision-making. Newhouse and colleagues[40(p36)] state that the EBP guidelines "stress a multidisciplinary approach and provide nurses with the structure and tools necessary to acquire EBP knowledge and skills, implement EBP changes in practice, and foster a stimulating, energizing and rewarding practice environment."

The conceptual model consists of a core of research and nonresearch evidence within the triad of professional nursing practice (practice, education, and research). EBP is impacted by internal organizational factors such as culture and environment and external factors including regulation and standards.[41]

The Johns Hopkins Nursing Evidence-Based Practice model is implemented using the PET process, an acronym for practice question, evidence, and translation. The process consists of 3 phases: practice question, evidence, and translation. The 3 phases include 18 prescriptive steps.[41] The practice question phase involves recruiting an interprofessional team, developing an EBP question and designating a leader. As part of the evidence phase, the team searches, appraises, summarizes, and synthesizes the literature. Recommendations are developed for change based on synthesis of the evidence. In the final phase, translation, the team determines the feasibility and appropriateness of the recommendations.

Translation theory and frameworks focus on "interrelationships and complex organizational dimensions" related to the translation of research or new knowledge into practice.[29(p32)] Rogers'[42] theory of diffusion of innovations, the foundation for many of the translation models will be described as an example of translation theory.

Rogers' Theory of Diffusion of Innovations

Rogers[43] diffusion of innovations model is one of the most popular models of organizational change used by nurses. The model provides a theoretic framework to support the implementation of EBP change. Diffusion is "the process by which an innovation is communicated through certain channels over time among the members of a social system."[42(p10)] The innovation decision is influenced by the kinds of communication channels and relationships, nature of the social system, characteristics of the decision-making unit and perceived characteristics of the innovation. The process as depicted in the model presents in a linear, unidirectional pattern that results in the adoption or rejection of the innovation.[44]

Rogers' theory describes a 5-step innovation decision process. Potential adopters of the innovation pass through 5 stages: knowledge, persuasion, decision, implementation, and confirmation. As they proceed through the stages, their understanding of the innovation might change and ultimately, they make a decision to either accept or reject the innovation.[44]

The knowledge stage involves the potential adopter becoming aware of the innovation and developing some understanding of how it functions.[44] In response to change or innovation, Rogers[43] identified 5 patterns of responses or adopter categories: innovators, early adopters, early majority, later majority, and laggards. Change often begins with the response by the innovators followed by the early adoptors, then early majority, later majority, and finally the laggards. An individual's pattern of response might vary depending on the change or innovation. As health care leaders, knowledge of the different patterns or categories of responses might be helpful to more effectively manage the change.[43]

The persuasion stage is the phase in the process in which the potential adopter forms a relatively favorable or unfavorable attitude toward the innovation.[44] In the knowledge stage, the potential adopter gains knowledge about the innovation; whereas, in the persuasion stage, they form attitudes toward the same. The relative advantage, compatibility, complexity, trialability, and observability are characteristics of the innovation or change that might impact the decision of those responsible for adopting the innovation. During the decision stage, the potential adopter participates in activities to accept or reject the innovation. The acceptance or rejection of the decision might not be permanent in this stage of the process.[44] In the implementation stage, the potential adopter initiates the process of implementing the innovation. Potential adopters might ask questions about the operationalization of the innovation. The final stage of the process is the confirmation stage. The potential adopters make permanent decisions to adopt or reject the innovation.

Table 3
Seven basic quality improvement tools most commonly used in health care

Tool or Technique Category	Tool Name	Description of Tool	Use the Tool When
Basic tools	Check sheet	• A simple check sheet is a structured, prepared form for collecting and analyzing data. This tool is generic and can be adapted for a wide variety of purposes.	• Observing and collecting data repeatedly by the same person or at the same location. • Collecting data on the frequency or patterns of events, problems, defects, etc. • Collecting data from a production process.
	Process flow diagram also called a process flowchart or process flow map	• Variations: micro flowchart, macro flowchart, top-down flowchart, detailed flowchart (also called process map, micro map, macro map, service map, or symbolic flowchart), deployment flowchart (also called down-across or cross-functional flowchart, swimlanes), several-leveled flowchart. • A process flow diagram or flowchart is a picture of the separate steps of a process in sequential order. • Elements may include sequence of actions or steps, materials or services entering or leaving the process (inputs and outputs), decisions that must be made, people involved in the process, time involved at each step and/or process measurements. • The process can be anything: a manufacturing process, an	• Developing an understanding of how a process is performed. • Studying a process for improvement. • Communicating to others how a process is performed. • Communicating between people involved with the same process. • Documenting a process. • Planning a project.

Fishbone diagram also called cause and effect diagram, or Ishikawa diagram or root cause analysis using the 5 whys.	administrative or service process, a project plan. This is a generic tool that can be adapted for a wide variety of purposes. • A fishbone diagram identifies many possible causes for an effect or problem. It can be used to structure a brainstorming session. It immediately sorts ideas into useful categories. ○ The 5 Whys: When a problem or error or defect occurs, it is critical to ask why. Asking why 5 times for each problem or defect identified allows you to get to the root cause of the problem or defect or error. If the root cause is not identified you may not find the right solution to the problem, defect, or error.	• Identifying possible causes for a problem, especially helpful if team's thinking becomes unproductive, dead end, or in a rut.
Run chart	A run chart is a line graph showing a process measurement on the vertical axis and the time on the horizontal axis. It is the simplest statistical tool. Often, a reference line shows the average of the data. • A graphical tool to monitor important process variables over time. • A helpful tool in identifying trends and cycles over time. • One of the most important tools for assessing the effectiveness of change.	• Monitoring a continuous variable over time. • Examining patterns, such as trends and cycles. • Conducting preliminary analysis to find obvious problems. • Collecting insufficient points of data to draw a control chart.

(continued on next page)

Table 3
(continued)

Tool or Technique Category	Tool Name	Description of Tool	Use the Tool When
Advanced statistical tools and techniques	Pareto chart also called Pareto diagram, Pareto analysis	• A Pareto chart is a bar graph. The lengths of the bars represent frequency or cost (time or money), and are arranged with longest bars on the left and the shortest to the right. In this way, the chart visually depicts which situations are more significant.	• Analyzing data about the frequency of problems or causes in a process. • Focusing on the most significant problem or cause; however, there are many problems or causes • Analyzing broad causes by looking at their specific components. • Communicating about the data with others.
	Control chart; also, Shewhart chart	• "A control chart is simply a run chart with statistically determined upper and lower limits drawn on either side of the process average that are determined by allowing a process to run untouched, then analyzed the results using a mathematical formula" (Walton, 19, p. 114). Data are plotted in time order. A control chart always has a central line for the average, an upper line for the upper control limit and a lower line for the lower control limit. These lines are determined from historical data. By comparing current data to these lines, you can draw conclusions about whether the process variation is consistent (in control) or is unpredictable (out of control, affected by special causes of variation).	• Studying how a process changes over time. • Analyzing patterns of process variation from special causes (nonroutine events) or common causes (built into the process). • Controlling ongoing processes by finding and correcting problems as they occur. • Predicting the expected range of outcomes from a process. • Determining whether a process is stable (in statistical control). • Determining whether the quality improvement project should aim to prevent specific process problems or to make fundamental changes to the process.

Histogram

- A histogram displays a frequency distribution of how often each different value in a set of data occurs. It is the most commonly used graph to show frequency distributions. Histograms look like a bar chart, but there are important differences between them.

- Examining data are numerical.
- Examining the shape of the data's distribution, especially when determining whether the output of a process is distributed approximately normally.
- Analyzing whether a process can meet the customer's requirements.
- Determining whether a process change has occurred from 1 time period to another.
- Determining whether the outputs of 2 or more processes are different.
- Communicating the distribution of data quickly and easily to others.

Data from Tague NR. The quality tool box. 2nd edition. Milwaukee (WI): Quality Press; 2005; and Christenbery TL. Evidence-based practice in nursing, foundations, skills, and roles. New York: Springer Publishing; 2018.

Adopters continue or discontinue the adoption and rejecters continue to reject or choose adoption.[43]

In their study, Gale and Schaffer[45] examined factors that influenced the organization's readiness to adopt or reject EBP changes and the differences in the perceptions of nurse managers and staff nurse about those factors. Roger's diffusion of innovations theory was used to provide background and guide the study. A nonrandomized group of nurse managers and staff nurses from 8 acute and critical care units completed the Evidence-Based Practice Changes Survey. Barriers to adopting EBP change included a lack of time, inadequate supplies and equipment, a perceived lack of support by nursing administration, and a lack of resources. The adoption of practice change should occur when the barriers are addressed by the organization.

QUALITY IMPROVEMENT TECHNIQUES AND TOOL BOX

Quality improvement tools drive the improvement scientific process that can lead to change. These tools help to predict conditions, performance, and process behavior. These tools allow us to collect and analyze data, quickly gaining process or system experience, which is important when there is an urgency to resolve a problem. Although there are many quality improvement tools, there are basically 7 tools most frequently used by quality improvement practitioners. The tools include a check sheet, process flow diagram or chart, cause and effect diagram (Ishikawa Diagram or fishbone), Pareto chart, histogram, and control chart.[46] **Table 3** lists the commonly used tools, briefly describing them and identifying when best to use them.

SUMMARY

As you read the selection of quality improvement projects in this issue of *Nursing Clinics of North America*, I would like you to think about the following questions:

- How did these health care providers translate new knowledge into action in their practice?
- Why are health care providers and organizations challenged when integrating new evidence or best practices?

REFERENCES

1. Baily MA, Bottrell MM, Lynn J, et al. Special report: the ethics of using QI methods to improve health care quality and safety. Hastings Cent Rep 2006;36(4):S1–40. Available at: https://muse-jhu-edu.proxy.library.vanderbilt.edu/article/201045/pdf. Accessed August 7, 2018.
2. Bolman LG, Deal T. Reframing organizations: artistry, choice, and leadership. Hoboken (NJ): John Wiley & Sons, Inc; 2017.
3. James B. Quality management for health care delivery. Chicago: The Hospital Research and Educational Trust of the American Hospital Association; 2004.
4. Perla RJ, Provost LP, Parry GJ. Seven propositions of the science of improvement: exploring foundations. Qual Manag Health Care 2013;22(3):170–86.
5. Langley GJ, Moen RD, Nolan KM, et al. The improvement guide: a practical approach to enhancing organizational performance. San Francisco (CA): Jossey-Bass Publishers; 1996.
6. Richardson WC, Berwick DM, Bisgard JC, et al. Crossing the quality chasm: a new health system for the 21st century. Washington, DC: National Academy Press; 2001.

7. Speroff T, James BC, Nelson EC, et al. Guidelines for appraisal and publication of PDSA quality improvement. Qual Manag Health Care 2004;13(1):33–9.
8. Lighter DE. Advanced performance improvement in health care: principles and methods. Sudbury (MA): Jones & Bartlett Publishers; 2011.
9. Deming WE. The new economics. Cambridge (MA): Massachusetts Institute of Technology; 1994.
10. Nolan T, Perla RJ, Provost L. Understanding variation. Qual Prog 2016;49(11):28.
11. Wheeler DJ. Understanding variation. Knoxville (TN): SPC Press, Inc; 1993.
12. Berwick DM. Controlling variation in health care: a consultation from Walter Shewhart. Med Care 1991;29(12):1212–25.
13. Lemire S, Christie CA, Inkelas M. The methods and tools of improvement science. In: Christie CA, Inkelas M, Lemire S, editors. Improvement science in evaluation: methods and uses: new directions for evaluation, number 153. Hoboken (NJ): Wiley Subscription Services, Inc; 2017. p. 23–33.
14. Health Foundation. Report: improvement science 2011. Available at: http://www.health.org.uk/publication/improvement-science.
15. Institute for Health Care Improvement (IHI). Science of improvement. 2018. Available at: http://www.ihi.org/about/Pages/ScienceofImprovement.aspx.
16. Langley GJ, Nolan KM, Nolan TW, et al. The improvement guide: a practical approach to enhancing organizational performance. 2nd edition. San Francisco (CA): Jossey-Bass Publishers; 2009.
17. Nelson EC, Batalden PB, Lazar JS, et al. Understanding clinical improvement: foundations of knowledge for change in health care systems. In: Nelson EC, Batalden PB, Lazar JS, editors. Practice-based learning and improvement: a clinical improvement action guide. Oakbrook Terrace (IL): Joint Commission Resources; 2007. p. 1–12.
18. Casartett D, Karlaswish JH, Sugarman J. Determining when quality improvement initiatives should be considered research, proposed criteria and potential implications. J Am Med Assoc 2009;283:2275–80.
19. Walsh K. Understanding what works – and why – in quality improvement: the need for theory-driven evaluation. Int J Qual Health Care 2007;19(2):57–9.
20. Vincent C, Taylor-Adams S, Stanhope N. Framework for analysing risk and safety in clinical medicine. BMJ 1998;316(7138):1154–7.
21. Jardali FE. Using data analysis frameworks for improving quality and safety. 6th Annual Conference on Quality Health Care. February 13, 2004.
22. Duke University School of Medicine. Contrasting QI and QA. 2016. Available at: http://patientsafetyed.duhs.duke.edu/module_a/introduction/contrasting_qi_qa.html. Accessed June 15, 2017.
23. NHS. First steps towards quality improvement: a simple guide to improving services. Published Unknown. Available at: http://webarchive.nationalarchives.gov.uk/20160805122504/http://www.nhsiq.nhs.uk/media/2591385/siguide.pdf. Accessed October 23, 2017.
24. Chalice R. Improving healthcare using Toyota lean production methods. 2nd edition. Milwaukee (WI): ASQ Quality Press; 2007.
25. HRSA. Improvement teams. 2016. Available at: http://www.hrsa.gov/quality/toolbox/508pdfs/improvementteams.pdf. Accessed November, 20, 2017. (in table).
26. Duke University School of Medicine. FADE. Published Unknown. 2016. Available at: http://patientsafetyed.duhs.duke.edu/module_d/why_healthcare.html. Accessed June 15, 2017. (in table).

27. Moen R, Norman C. Evolution of the PDSA cycle. 2006. Available at: http://www.uoc.cw/financesite/images/stories/NA01_Moen_Norman_fullpaper.pdf. Accessed August 7, 2018.
28. Liker J, Franz JK. The Toyota way to continuous improvement: linking strategy and operational excellence to achieve superior performance. New York: McGraw Hill; 2011.
29. White KM. The science of translation and major frameworks. In: White KM, Dudley-Brown S, Terhaar MF, editors. Translation of evidence into nursing and health care. 2nd edition. New York: Springer Publishing Company; 2016.
30. Kanter MH, Schottinger J, Whittaker J. A model for implementing evidence-based practices more quickly. NEJM Catalyst; 2017.
31. Schuster MA, McGlynn EA, Brooke RH. How good is the quality of health care in the United States? Milbank Q 1998;76(4):517–63.
32. Agency for Health Care Policy and Research. Translating research into practice. RFA: HS-99-003. January 8, 1999. Available at: https://grants.nih.gov/grants/guide/rfa-files/RFA-HS-99-003.html.
33. Agency for Healthcare Research and Quality (AHRQ). Translating research into practice (TRIP-II) fact sheet 2001. Available at: http://ahrq.gov/research/trip2fac.htm.
34. Farquhar CM, Stryer D, Slutsky J. Translating research into practice: the future ahead. International Journal for Quality in Health Care 2002;14(3):233–49.
35. Institute for Healthcare Improvement. 5 Million Lives Campaign. Getting started kit: sustainability and spread. Cambridge (MA): 2008. Available at: http://www.ihi.org/Engage/Initiatives/Completed/5MillionLivesCampaign/Pages/default.aspx.
36. Titler MG, Kleiber C, Steelman V, et al. The Iowa model of evidence-based practice to promote quality care. Crit Care Nurs Clin North Am 2001;13(4):497–509.
37. Melnyk BM, Fineout-Overholt E. Evidence-based practice in nursing & healthcare. 3rd edition. New York: Wolters Kluwer; 2015.
38. McEwen M, Wills EM. Theoretical basis for nursing. 4th edition. New York: Wolters Kluwer/Lippincott Williams & Wilkins; 2014.
39. Melnyk BM, Fineout-Overholt E. Making the case for evidence-based practice and cultivating the spirit of inquiry. In: Melnyk BM, Fineout-Overholt E, editors. Evidence-based practice in nursing and healthcare: a guide to best practice. 2nd edition. Philadelphia: Lippincott Williams & Wilkins; 2011. p. 3–24.
40. Newhouse R, Dearbolt S, Poe S, et al. Evidence-based practice. A practical approach to implementation. J Nurs Adm 2005;35(1):35–40.
41. Dearholt SL, White K, Newhouse RP, et al. Educational strategies to develop evidence-based practice mentors. J Nurses Staff Dev 2008;24(2):53–9.
42. Rogers EM. Diffusion of innovations. 5th edition. New York: The Free Press; 2003.
43. Rogers E. Diffusion of innovations. 4th edition. New York: The Free Press; 1995.
44. Tiffany CR, Lutjens LRJ. Planned change theories for nursing: review, analysis, and implications. Thousand Oaks (CA): Sage Publications, Inc; 1998.
45. Gale BVP, Schaffer MA. Organizational readiness for evidence-based practice. J Nurs Adm 2009;39(2):91–7.
46. Tague NR. The quality toolbox, vol. 600. Milwaukee (WI): ASQ Quality Press; 2005.

Chart It to Stop It

Failure Modes and Effect Analysis for the Reporting of Workplace Aggression

Gordon Lee Gillespie, PhD, DNP, RN, CEN, CNE, CPEN, PHCNS-BC[a],*,
Treasa 'Susie' Leming-Lee, DNP, MSN, RN[b]

KEYWORDS

- Workplace violence • Emergency department • Safety committee
- Quality improvement

KEY POINTS

- Priority of actions needs to be assigned to reducing the failure modes for notifying the emergency department director about occurrences of workplace aggression.
- Workplace aggression prevention efforts led by a workplace aggression committee have potential to overcome many of the failure modes and causes identified in this study.
- Failure modes and effect analysis is an effective process to identify the tasks for and failure modes, causes, and effects of reporting workplace aggression.

Workplace aggression (WPA) is enacted against health care workers at an alarming rate. The Occupational Safety and Health Administration estimates the prevalence of WPA in the health care and social assistance sector at 7.8 per 10,000 full-time workers from 2002 to 2013 compared with approximately 1.8 per 10,000 full-time workers for all private industries combined.[1] A challenge to obtaining reliable prevalence data in health care settings is the lack of WPA reporting. Several reasons have been reported to explain this lack of reporting; however, none are focused on the reporting process itself. The purpose of this article is to describe the process for WPA reporting and the potential failures for this process in a pediatric emergency department.

BACKGROUND

WPA is a behavior perceived as offensive or threatening (eg, verbal abuse, sexual abuse) as well as a threat of physical violence and assaults.[2] WPA in a pediatric setting

Disclosure Statement: This study was funded by the Robert Wood Johnson Foundation.
[a] Institute for Nursing Research and Scholarship, College of Nursing, University of Cincinnati, PO Box 21-0038, Cincinnati, OH 45221-0038, USA; [b] Vanderbilt University School of Nursing, 461 21st Avenue South, 216 Godchaux Hall, Nashville, TN 37240, USA
* Corresponding author.
E-mail address: gordon.gillespie@uc.edu

Nurs Clin N Am 54 (2019) 21–32
https://doi.org/10.1016/j.cnur.2018.10.004

is not new. McAneney and Shaw in their seminal cross-sectional study of pediatric emergency department directors (n = 44) in 1994 found WPA to be an emerging problem.[3] At that time, about half of the sample had already begun confiscating weapons from patients and visitors. This burden of WPA has only increased over the last 25 years. More recently, Shaw studied perceptions of safety and fear in 191 employees working in a pediatric emergency department.[4] She found concerns for safety and fear were realized due to agitated patients and visitors, presence of weapons brought into the emergency department, and lack of security presence. Gillespie, Gates, Miller, and Howard found a similar finding in that WPA management was a problem in the pediatric emergency department particularly in relation to availability, responsiveness, and perceived effectiveness of security officers.[5]

Multiple reasons account for the WPA reporting/underreporting in health care settings. Arnetz and colleagues[6] found the prevalence of WPA underreporting to be as high as 88%. Although formal reporting was infrequent, the researchers discovered that many victims of WPA did use informal means for WPA reporting such as verbally informing their supervisors and calling a Compliance Hotline. Reasons for underreporting included not having enough time to complete a report, reporting not leading to changes, and WPA not being important enough to report. Similar findings were discussed by Gillespie and colleagues and Sato and coleagues.[7,8] In addition, these researchers identified the perceived normalization of WPA, lack of administrator support, and lack of intention to cause harm by the aggressor as factors explaining WPA underreporting. Despite the prevalence of and reasons for WPA reporting/underreporting, a complete account of WPA occurrences is crucial to develop effective interventions for the future prevention of WPA.[6] A necessary next step to address WPA is identifying the process for WPA reporting and recognizing strategies to overcome potential failures in the process.

METHODS

This quality improvement study used a failure modes and effect analysis (FMEA) design to describe the WPA reporting process and potential failures for this process. This study was deemed not human subjects research by the authors' affiliated Institutional Review Boards.

FMEA has been in use for more than 50 years[9] and described as "a systematic, proactive method for evaluating a process to identify where and how it might fail and to assess the relative impact of different failures, in order to identify the parts of the process that are most in need of change" (para 1).[10] The FMEA design focuses on identifying the steps in the process as well as the failure modes, causes, and effects. FMEA has been used frequently to address other health care processes including risk identification and injury prevention,[11] medical emergency response teams for cardiac arrest,[12] blood transfusion in pediatrics,[13] fibrinolytic administration for acute myocardial infarction,[14] communication failures,[15] and process of emergency care.[16]

The FMEA method used in this study was adapted from the Institute for Healthcare Improvement and Schriefer and Leonard.[10,17] The method includes the following:

1. Selecting a process to evaluate with FMEA.
2. Recruit a multidisciplinary team.
3. Have the team meet together to list all of the steps in the process.
4. Have the team list failure modes and causes.
5. For each failure mode, have the team assign a numeric value for likelihood of occurrence, likelihood of detection, and severity.

6. Evaluate the results.
7. Use risk profile number to plan improvement efforts.

Setting

This study was conducted at a pediatric teaching hospital in the Midwest United States. The emergency department where the data were collected treats approximately 100,000 patients per year. Between 3:00 AM and 10:59 AM, staffing is at the lowest number for the day with approximately 11 to 13 patient services employees. Between 3:00 PM and 10:59 PM, staffing is at the highest for the day with approximately 32 to 37 patient services employees. Staffing varies by day of week and time of day based on trends in patient volume. A 30-day prevalence for WPA from a previous convenience sample of 101 workers in this setting reflected 128 occurrences of verbal abuse, 3 occurrences of sexual abuse, 43 occurrences of physical threats, and 59 occurrences of assaults. Although the prevalence may be remarkably high, a large portion of these events were not formally reported into the hospital's electronic safety management system.

Sample

During a walkthrough assessment of the pediatric emergency department, employees were solicited to answer questions about the WPA reporting process. Employees solicited to participate represented several disciplines and multiple areas of the emergency department (ie, lobby, triage, trauma bay, treatment area). Employees recruited were working during 1 of 2 different days proximal to the 7:00 AM shift change. Interviews were conducted during this time period to reduce the chance the interviews would cause a delay in patient care.

Procedures for FMEA Assessment

Interviews with 10 pediatric emergency department employees were conducted. Potential participants were informed of the study purpose and their rights to voluntarily participate or decline participation. All employees solicited opted to participate. With permission and often at their request, interviews were conducted at their workstations in the nursing station or at the security desk. Also, interviews were conducted during their regular shift just before or just after the 7:00 AM shift change. During the interviews, other employees would join the conversation and provide affirmation or additional context to the information provided by the primary respondents. The interview questions were as follows:[10]

1. What are the steps of the process for WPA reporting?
2. What could go wrong in the process? [failure modes]
3. Why would the failure happen? [failure causes]
4. What are the potential consequences of failures? [failure effects]

During the interviews, handwritten notes were taken to document the reporting process and potential failures. A summary of the process and potential failures were verified with respondents at the end of the interviews.

Based on discussions with respondents and identified failure modes, causes, and effects, numeric values were assigned for the likelihood of occurrence, likelihood of detection, and severity. Likelihood of a failure mode occurring was scored using a Likert scale ranging from 1 (very unlikely to occur) to 10 (very likely to occur). Likelihood of detecting a failure mode was scored using a Likert scale ranging from 1 (very likely to be detected) to 10 (very unlikely to be detected). Severity of the failure mode was rated using a Likert scale ranging from 1 (very unlikely that harm will occur) to 10 (very likely that severe harm will occur). Finally, a risk profile number was calculated by multiplying together the scores for the likelihood of occurrence, likelihood of detection, and severity.

The findings then were discussed and verified with the emergency department's Professional Education Council who also made recommendations on next steps. This council served as the multidisciplinary team throughout the project period. Council membership included registered nurses, a respiratory therapist, paramedic, patient care assistant, child life specialist, and clinical manager.

RESULTS

Ten employees formally participated in the interview questions. Half (n = 5) of the respondents were registered nurses. Remaining respondents were 2 security officers, 1 nurse educator, 1 patient care assistant, and 1 registration clerk.

Process for WPA Reporting

A synthesis of the interviews reflected 7 tasks to occur following an occurrence of WPA: (1) contact security, (2) contact police, (3) contact clinical manager, (4) notify emergency department director, (5) call safety hotline, (6) complete electronic safety form, and (7) complete paper safety form. The process was nonlinear and not all steps were relevant for each occurrence of WPA. These tasks are displayed in **Fig. 1**. In the next section, the failure modes, causes, and effects for these tasks are described.

Failure Modes, Causes, and Effects

Task 1: contact security
Following an occurrence of WPA, the employee receiving or witnessing the aggression is supposed to contact a security officer. Respondents indicated they did not routinely contact security, particularly if the aggression was verbal abuse. By not contacting security for all WPA including verbal abuse, protective services support would not be in place should the aggression escalate to physical assault. Without security's presence

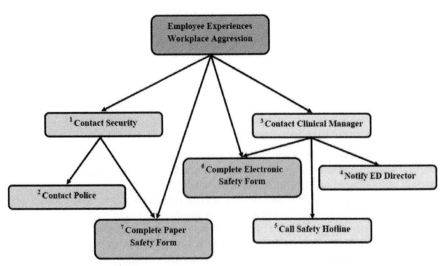

Fig. 1. Process for reporting an occurrence of workplace aggression.

and intervention, the outcome of the WPA could be worsened. These failure modes, causes, and effects led to a risk priority number of 141 (**Table 1**).

Task 2: contact police

When WPA was perceived to be significant (eg, not effectively managed by security), the security officer would request police support. Respondents posited an inconsistency for when security officers would contact police. It was not clear to them at what point the situation was deemed unresolvable or escalating beyond safe management. In other instances of WPA, employees said they would contact police themselves "just in case things went south [became worse]." This inconsistency in police usage could lead to ineffective police intervention or delay police response when another WPA event occurs. These failure modes, causes, and effects led to a risk priority number of 147.

Task 3: contact clinical manager

In addition to contacting security following an occurrence of WPA, the employee is supposed to contact the clinical manager for support, if one is on duty. Failure to contact the clinical manager depended on the shift and particular clinical manager on duty. The shift least likely to contact the clinical manager about WPA was night shift. Respondents explained a clinical manager had other duties when they were on shift and may not see the clinical manager until the end of the shift. By the end of the shift, the respondents had already forgotten about the WPA unless the event was a significant threat or assault. A couple respondents did not feel supported during a previous WPA report and opted to not report future WPA occurrences if the same clinical manager was on duty. This lack of reporting prevents employees in general to receive the necessary administrative support following acts of WPA. These failure modes, causes, and effects led to a risk priority number of 144.

Task 4: notify emergency department director

At the end of each shift, the clinical manager on duty is supposed to notify the emergency department director about negative events including WPA. An advantage of this step is department leadership routinely being made aware of WPA contemporaneously when the events occurred. Failures to this process occurred when employees did not contact the clinical manager and thus the clinical manager was not able to notify the emergency department director. When a clinical manager was not on duty, employees could notify the charge nurse who would be accountable to notify the director. However, charge nurses inconsistently notified the director. Without the director being made aware as to the prevalence of the problem, additional resources such as increased staffing and security officer presence would not be prioritized. These failure modes, causes, and effects led to a risk priority number of 360.

Task 5: call safety hotline

At the end of each shift, the clinical manager on duty also is supposed to leave a voicemail message on the safety hotline. This safety hotline recording can be reviewed by the hospital administration, risk management, and other key leaders. In the absence of the clinical manager, employees could notify the charge nurse who could leave the message on the safety hotline. As previously written, when employees did not notify the clinical manager or charge nurse about the WPA event, then the report could not be left on the safety hotline. Another failure in the process was that employees could not articulate what happens to their reports once they were disseminated to the safety hotline. Similar to the effects for not notifying the director, additional resources would not be prioritized to the emergency department. Of greater

Table 1
Failure modes and effects analysis for WPA reporting

Processes	Failure Modes	Failure Causes	Failure Effects	Likelihood of Occurrence (1–10)	Likelihood of Detection (1–10)	Severity (1–10)	Risk Priority Number	Actions to Reduce Occurrence of Failure
Contact security	Security not called	Verbal abuse No intent by aggressor to cause harm	Aggression escalates without security intervention	7	9	4	141	Security rounds department to identify aggression events Education on interventions that could be put into place for WPA that is not intentional
Contact police	Police not called Police called for minor events	Security perceives they can manage the event without assistance Police could respond faster than security Security perceived as not effective	Ineffective use of police Police not available for another call	7	3	7	147	Develop policy on when police to be contacted Set expectations for security effectiveness
Contact clinical manager	Clinical manager not notified	Not on shift Forgot to notify by end of shift	No support by clinical manager whether occurrence reported	8	9	2	144	Clinical manager rounds and asks about occurrences Clinical manager follows-up with employees who report events

Process step	Failure mode	Effect	Severity	Occurrence	Detection	RPN	Recommended actions
Notify ED director	ED director not informed of events; Clinical manager not informed of event; Nothing will change if director notified	Director not aware of prevalence of problem; Decisions to prevent future WPA not based on reliable data	8	9	5	360	ED director rounds and asks about occurrences; ED director follows-up with employees who report events; Submit notification to a single corporate email (eg, WPV-reporting@___.org) with simultaneous delivery to upper administration, ED director, risk management, and security; Communicate efforts to prevent future WPA
Call safety hotline	Employees do not notify clinical manager or charge nurse; Clinical manager or charge nurse forget to call hotline number	Employees not aware what happens after a report is made to safety hotline; Clinical manager or charge nurse too busy to call hotline number; Decisions to prevent future WPA not based on reliable data	8	3	5	120	Clinical manager or charge nurse rounds and asks about occurrences; Incoming clinical manager or charge nurse asks outgoing person if call made to safety hotline

(continued on next page)

Table 1
(continued)

Processes	Failure Modes	Failure Causes	Failure Effects	Likelihood of Occurrence (1–10)	Likelihood of Detection (1–10)	Severity (1–10)	Risk Priority Number	Actions to Reduce Occurrence of Failure
Complete electronic safety form	Form not filled out, Form incomplete	Takes too long to complete form, Too many required fields on form, Not suitable for visitor aggression, WPA is normalized	Decisions to prevent future WPA not based on reliable data, Clinical manager will need to complete form for employee	9	6	5	270	Revise electronic form to have fewer required fields, Revise electronic form to allow reports on visitors, Education that WPA is not part of the job and should not be tolerated
Complete paper safety form	Form not filled out, Form incomplete	Not suitable for visitor aggression, Forms not available, Forms not collected regularly, Verbal abuse not severe enough to report	Decisions to prevent future WPA not based on reliable data	4	3	5	60	Restock forms daily, Have clinical manager collect forms each shift, Education on importance of reporting

Abbreviation: ED, emergency department.

consequence, without the safety hotline notification, the only channel for higher administration to become aware of the WPA prevalence would be through the director. These failure modes, causes, and effects led to a risk priority number of 280.

Task 6: complete electronic safety form

Employees consistently reported they were expected to formally report all WPA occurrences via the hospital's electronic safety form. An advantage of the electronic safety form is the in-depth nature of the report and use of prefilled content that could be "checked" while still allowing for a narrative description of the event. A burden of the electronic safety form was the time required to complete the report (eg, 20 minutes) and requirement to enter patient identifiers. When events did not lead to a physical injury, employees reported the system was too cumbersome and time consuming to complete. When WPA was enacted by a visitor, there was no way in the electronic system to note this other than the open field at the end. Employees also were concerned about the electronic safety form being used to flag a patient as aggressive when the WPA was enacted not by the patient but a patient's visitor. When the electronic safety form was not completed and the clinical manager became aware of the WPA event, the clinical manager would complete the form on the employee's behalf. This surrogate data entry could lead to discrepancies in documentation between the documented and actual event. The lack of reporting coupled with the potential for inaccurate data could lead to WPA prevention decisions made on unreliable findings. These failure modes, causes, and effects led to a risk priority number of 120.

Task 7: complete paper safety form

Employees were given the option to complete a paper safety form in lieu of the electronic safety form. An advantage to the paper safety form was it takes about 2 minutes to complete. Information requested on the form was a patient label, description of the event, time/date of the event, and name of person completing the report. The paper safety form then is deposited into a locked box available in multiple locations throughout the department. Each weekday morning, the boxes were emptied and forms given to the clinical manager on duty. A failure observed to this task was that the supply of forms was empty in several locations. Employees indicated that unless the occurrence was severe, they would not walk to another area of the department to retrieve and complete the form. Another barrier to completing the form was the requirement for the patient label. When aggression was enacted by a visitor, the employees may not have known who the visitor was visiting, thus they opted to not report the WPA. A primary failure for reporting WPA with both the paper and electronic safety forms was that the perception security consistently completed these forms and their information would only be duplicative and not needed. These failure modes, causes, and effects led to a risk priority number of 60.

DISCUSSION

The purpose of this quality improvement study to describe the process for WPA reporting and potential failures was achieved. For the process of WPA reporting, there were 7 related but nonlinear tasks to perform following an act of WPA enacted by a patient or visitor. Multiple potential failures to the process were posited. Based on an assessment of the failure modes, causes, and effects; likelihood of occurrence; likelihood of detection; and severity, a risk priority number was calculated. Risk priority numbers ranged from a low of 60 for completing a paper form to a high of 360 for notifying the emergency department director.

Based on the findings (risk priority numbers), priority needs to be assigned to reducing the failure modes for notifying the emergency department director. On a collaborative discussion with the emergency department's interdisciplinary Professional Education Council, this focus was affirmed. Also, it was agreed that a predominant reason for not notifying the director was the perception that nothing would change even if WPA was reported. This determination is consistent with the published literature.[6–8,18] A key action to address failure modes and failure causes is sharing findings and improvements for WPA management with employees.[19] As employees become aware of organizational efforts to improve their work environment based on their data, they may be more likely to increase their WPA reporting. This increased reporting also may benefit failure modes for completing an electronic and/or paper safety forms.

Completing an electronic safety form had the second highest risk priority number. Revising the electronic safety form can be considered in order to meet the needs of risk management, department leadership, and upper administration while reducing the reporting burden for employees. Arnetz and colleagues[20] concluded stakeholder input is necessary when designing or revising the reporting system. Considerations for the system can include preferred content, format, and use of the reports. A particular remedy is the ability to complete a report without entering patient information (ie, reporting visitor WPA).

WPA prevention efforts led by a WPA committee have potential to overcome many of the failure modes and causes identified in this study. A WPA committee could coordinate education on WPA not being part of the job, WPA should not be tolerated or accepted, unintentional WPA is still WPA, and WPA needs to be reported. The American Organization of Nurse Executives, Emergency Nurses Association, and Occupational Safety and Health Administration also recommended the use of a WPA committee to provide strategic direction on WPA prevention and management, ongoing assessment, and evaluation of achieving program goals.[1,19,21] Additional actions a WPA committee at the current pediatric emergency department could lead are establishing a WPA policy clarifying when police would be notified by security; under what circumstances staff could directly contact police for support; making WPA reporting mandatory; process for regular rounding by charge nurses, clinical managers, and emergency department director to inquire about WPA events; and the frequency to restock paper safety forms (ie, daily).

Limitations

There were 2 factors limiting the findings for this quality improvement study. First, selection bias may have occurred by how the respondents were identified. For example, the perceptions of the employees available for interviews proximal to the 7:00 AM shift change may be different from the perceptions of employees at 7:00 PM. This limitation was lessened given that more than half of the employees at the study site worked 12-hour shifts and either started or ended their shifts at 7:00 AM. Second, response bias may have occurred with respondents providing misleading information. This limitation was not likely to have occurred, because all respondents along with their coworkers who joined the interviews provided consistent information, thus legitimizing the study findings.

SUMMARY

FMEA was an effective process to identify the tasks for and failure modes, causes, and effects of reporting WPA. Efforts to reduce failure modes can be coordinated by an interdisciplinary WPA committee. Focusing actions to failure modes and causes for the notification of the emergency department director and completion of an electronic safety form can garner the greatest improvement in overall risk for WPA reporting. Future quality improvement efforts can explore the impact of a WPA policy and formation of a WPA committee to reduce the prevalence and increase the reporting of WPA.

ACKNOWLEDGMENTS

The authors wish to thank Terri Crutcher, DNP, RN and Jennifer Mattei, DNP, RN, CPN for their support during the conduct of this study.

REFERENCES

1. Occupational Safety and Health Administration. Workplace violence in health-care: understanding the challenge. Washington, DC: Author; 2015.
2. National Institute for Occupational Safety and Health. Occupational hazards in hospitals. Cincinnati (OH): National Institute for Occupational Safety and Health; 2002.
3. McAneney CM, Shaw KN. Violence in the pediatric emergency department. Ann Emerg Med 1994;23(6):1248–51.
4. Shaw J. Staff perceptions of workplace violence in a pediatric emergency department. Work 2015;51(1):39–49.
5. Gillespie GL, Gates DM, Miller M, et al. Emergency department workers' perceptions of security officers' effectiveness during violent events. Work 2012;42(1): 21–7.
6. Arnetz JE, Hamblin L, Ager J, et al. Underreporting of workplace violence: comparison of self-report and actual documentation of hospital incidents. Workplace Health Saf 2015;63(5):200–10.
7. Sato K, Wakabayashi T, Kiyoshi-Teo H, et al. Factors associated with nurses' reporting of patients' aggressive behavior: a cross-sectional survey. Int J Nurs Stud 2013;50:1368–76.
8. Gillespie GL, Leming-Lee T, Crutcher T, et al. Chart it to stop it: a quality improvement study to increase the reporting of workplace aggression. J Nurs Care Qual 2016;31(3):254–61.
9. Jerson T, Myers R. Saturn S-IC stage operational experience. New York: Society of Automotive Engineers; 1968.
10. Institute for Healthcare Improvement. Failure modes and effects analysis (FMEA) tool. 2018. Available at: http://www.ihi.org/resources/Pages/Tools/Failure ModesandEffectsAnalysisTool.aspx. Accessed November 20, 2018.
11. Paparella S. Failure mode and effects analysis: a useful tool for risk identification and injury prevention. J Emerg Nurs 2007;33(4):367–71.
12. Chan ML, Spertus JA, Tang F, et al. Missed opportunities in use of medical emergency teams prior to in-hospital cardiac arrest. Am Heart J 2016;177:87–95.
13. Dehnavieh R, Ebrahimipour H, Molavi-Taleghani Y, et al. Proactive risk assessment of blood transfusion process, in pediatric emergency, using the health care failure mode and effects analysis (HFMEA). Glob J Health Sci 2015;7(1): 322–31.
14. Jensen JL, Walker M, Denike D, et al. Paramedic myocardia infarction care with fibrinolytics: a process map and hazard analysis. Prehosp Emerg Care 2013; 17(4):429–34.

15. Mojica E, Izarzugaza E, Gonzalez M, et al. Elaboration of a risk map in a paediatric emergency department of a teaching hospital. Emerg Med J 2016;33(10): 684–9.
16. Bagnasco A, Tubino B, Piccotti E, et al. Identifying and correcting communication failures among health professionals working in the emergency department. Int Emerg Nurs 2013;21(3):168–72.
17. Schriefer J, Leonard MS. Patient safety and quality improvement: an overview of QI. Pediatr Rev 2012;33(8):353–60.
18. Enam GH, Alimohammadi H, Sadrabad AZ, et al. Workplace violence against residents in emergency department and reasons for not reporting them: a cross sectional study. Emergency 2018;6(1):e7.
19. American Organization of Nurse Executives and Emergency Nurses Association. Toolkit for mitigating violence in the workplace. n.d. Available at: http://www.aone. org/resources/final_toolkit.pdf. Accessed November 20, 2018.
20. Arnetz JE, Hamblin L, Ager J, et al. Using database reports to reduce workplace violence: Perceptions of hospital stakeholders. Work 2015;51(1):51–9.
21. American Organization of Nurse Executives and Emergency Nurses Association. AONE guiding principles: mitigating violence in the workplace. 2015. Available at: http://www.aone.org/resources/mitigating-workplace-violence.pdf. Accessed November 20, 2018.

The Effects of a Targeted History Question on Patient-Triage Nurse Communication

Kristyn C. Huffman, DNP, RN, AGACNP-BC

KEYWORDS

- Emergency department • Triage • QuickLook • Fast track • Past medical history
- Nursing communication

KEY POINTS

- Past medical history is an integral part of triage in emergency departments.
- Triage is being streamlined to increase patient throughput, which leads to triage discrepancies.
- QuickLook, as a modified triage process, does not account for past medical history.
- Pertinent past medical history can be assessed during triage without prolonging total triage times.

A quality improvement (QI) project sought to improve patient placement between fast track (FT) and the emergency department (ED) in an urban Southern Arizona hospital. The modified triage process at this hospital, known as QuickLook (QL), limits the information received by the triage nurse by omitting patient past medical history (PMH). This article discusses how the QI project sought to improve patient to triage nurse communication by educating nurses to ask a targeted history (TH) question: a question to gather concise PMH information related to the patient's chief complaint. This TH question was worded as "Have you been treated for [chief complaint] before?" The data collection process and results regarding Emergency Severity Index (ESI) scores, triage times, and nursing compliance rates are reviewed, along with recommendations for improving communication during triage.

INTRODUCTION

Visits to EDs in the United States continue to climb upward of 130 million each year, leading to overcrowding, triage discrepancies, and numerous patient adverse events.[1–3] FTs have been implemented in EDs to address overcrowding and increase

Disclosure Statement: The author has no financial interests to disclose.
University Of Arizona College of Nursing, 1305 N Martin Avenue, Tucson, AZ 85721, USA
E-mail address: khuffman@email.arizona.edu

patient throughput by expediting treatment for low-acuity patients.[4,5] Patients are triaged in the ED using the ESI, a standardized triage algorithm supported by the Agency for Healthcare Research and Quality for use in EDs throughout the United States.[6] Triage nurses assign patients an acuity level ranging from 1 to 5, with 1 signifying the patient needs immediate life-saving interventions and 5 signifying no emergent interventions are needed.[6] Nearly 80% of the EDs in the United States have implemented FTs as treatment areas for low-acuity patients,[7] typically treating ESI Levels 4 and 5.

QuickLook

A major academic hospital in Southern Arizona uses a modified triage process known as QL. This modified triage is intended to increase patient throughput by setting a 3-minute time limit for the triage registered nurse (TRN) to complete triage and assign an ESI acuity. QL is a single navigation page built into the hospital's electronic health record (EHR). The TRN follows the ESI algorithm and completes the QL navigation page to collect patient data on the chief complaint, last menstrual period, allergies, vital signs, pain, Glasgow Coma Scale score, height/weight, recent travel for Ebola screening, diabetes status, and smoking history. The TRN then writes a one-line triage note in the EHR and completes QL by assigning an ESI level to the patient. QL does not prompt the triage nurse to ask the patient about their PMH, beyond diabetes and smoking status. The collection of PMH is eliminated from this modified triage process to keep average triage times to 3 minutes or less. The patient is then placed in either FT or the main ED for treatment.

LITERATURE REVIEW
Past Medical History in Triage

A literature search was conducted using the databases PubMed, CINAHL, and Google Scholar for articles containing the key search terms: "triage," "emergency department," "fast track," "assessment," and "PMH." Variations of the search term "quicklook" were used, but no applicable literature was found. The search was limited to English language studies published within the last 10 years (2006–2016). Studies considered for inclusion specifically addressed the triage process within the ED and pertained only to adult subjects. The publications that were excluded lacked statistical significance or evidence-based information. In total, 10 publications were reviewed and evaluated for the purposes of the QI project. This article focuses on the publications specifically pertaining to PMH in triage, which are reviewed in Appendix 1 and the following text.

Half of included literature demonstrated health care professionals regard PMH as an integral part of triage.[8–12] When examining the role of PMH in triage, it is important to identify its relevance to critically ill patients in EDs.[4] A retrospective study of patients with myocardial infarction (MI) in the ED requiring percutaneous coronary intervention found that 57% had a history of hypertension, 38% had a history of hyperlipidemia, and 9% had a prior MI.[9] Four studies specifically commented on the important role PMH has in the triage decision-making process for patients with MI.[8,9,11,13] A questionnaire sent to Emergency Nursing Association members showed that 429 out of 430 respondents "strongly agree" with PMH being an important part of the triage process.[10] Almost all respondents reported their facility required PMH to be assessed during triage.[10] Castner[10] recommends these findings be used to prioritize the clinical data nurses obtain during triage. Wolf[12] used simulated patient scenarios to examine triage nurse accuracy for assigning ESI scores to patients. Nurses were found to have an ESI accuracy of 48% to 69% for all simulated scenarios.[12] Assigning an inaccurate ESI score was directly attributed to the TRN ignoring vital signs, not using a working diagnosis, and not asking the patient about their PMH.[12]

Gaps in Literature

Several of the included studies demonstrate triage is more heavily influenced by subjective nurse-related factors.[8,14,15] Current literature describes the many influencing factors of triage, but there are still many variables that need to be researched. Available research has discussed explanations for how nursing and facility variables affect ESI acuity scores. However, almost no literature exists regarding the effects of specific questions asked and the subsequent information obtained during triage. Although there are several studies that identify PMH as a necessary part of the triage process, only one study specifically addressed the effects of PMH on triage accuracy.[12] Considering this study directly attributed 50% of triage error to a lack of PMH, Wolf[12] suggests further research be conducted on the importance of PMH in triage.

PURPOSE

The original purpose of this QI project was to integrate a TH question into the QL triage navigation page to increase effective patient-to-nurse communication in the ED. The primary purpose of this project remained consistent, but alterations to the original plan were necessary directly before starting implementation. It was found the EHR could not be altered to include the TH question, as originally planned, after the author received final permission to begin implementation from the appropriate hospital personnel. Because of this misunderstanding, this QI project's plan was changed days before implementation to incorporate educating TRNs to ask the TH question and then write patient responses directly into the triage note. The author then received additional permission to access all necessary triage notes to facilitate data collection for this project.

METHODS

This QI project was guided by the Plan-Do-Study-Act (PDSA) model of change to implement a change, the TH question, to the current ED triage process. A TH question is defined as a single-sentence question about the patient's chief complaint, prompting the patient to respond to the TRN with specific and concise information about his or her PMH. TRNs were instructed to ask patients the TH question: "Have you been treated for [chief complaint] before?" For example, for a patient with a chief complaint of chest pain, the TRN should ask "Have you been treated for chest pain before?" TRNs were instructed to write an acceptable form of TH into the triage note along with the patient's response, used later during EHR audits for tracking purposes. Acceptable forms of TH in triage notes included: targeted history, target history, TH, and THx.

Design

Rouen[16] defines QI projects as the systematic collection of data to evaluate and improve quality and safety outcomes within health care. This descriptive design QI project aimed to use data-based methods to improve health care outcomes.[17] The implementation of this QI project was guided by the PDSA method, a four-step process that allows for rapid implementation and assessment of an intervention within a short timeframe.[18] This QI project consisted of two PDSA cycles, each over a 2-week period, to facilitate the implementation of the TH question into QL. Step 1 of PDSA Cycle 1 (C1), *plan*, consisted of planning the logistics of the proposed change and obtaining all necessary permissions for implementation. Step 2, *do*, involved testing the TH question on a small scale.[18] Step 2 for each cycle was completed within a single ED, each over the 2-week timeframe previously mentioned. Step 3, *study*, involved conducting chart audits of the EHR for data collection and analysis once Step 2 was completed.[18] Information learned from PDSA C1 was disseminated in Step 4, *act*, where the original plan was refined based on findings from previous steps in the cycle.[18]

Information learned from PDSA C1 was then integrated into PDSA Cycle 2 (C2), a second 2-week PDSA cycle. Step 1 of C2, *plan*, was changed to provide triage nurses with a more thorough 5-minute in-service, clarifying how to integrate the TH question into the triage interview. Triage nurses were also provided with more frequent reminders, based on feedback from C1, to ask the TH question. The processes of Step 2 (C2), *do*, and *Step* 3 (C2), *study*, were repeated from C1. Step 4 of PDSA C2, *act*, involved the dissemination of project findings to stakeholders at the facility.

Secondary purposes of this QI project were satisfied through qualitative methods. Discourse analysis, used by sociolinguists to understand the mechanisms and structures of conversations,[19] guided the analysis of transcripts translated from audio recordings between stakeholders and the author. Stakeholders important to this QI project were triage nurses, nurse practitioners, and attending physicians in the facility's ED. Stakeholders were interviewed with open-ended questions (Appendices 2 and 3) about their perceptions of the TH question at the beginning and end stages of each PDSA cycle. Participants for interviews were recruited through convenience sampling conducted within the triage and FT treatment areas. The author acknowledges that although convenience sampling is not the preferred sampling method for collecting the greatest amount of information,[19] it was the most practical form of sampling for this project.

Setting

This project took place in the ED of an urban level 1 trauma center in Southern Arizona. The ED is separated by pediatric versus adult, with a 40-bed adult-only treatment area and three adult-only triage rooms. Triage is staffed with two to three triage nurses and an attending physician. FT is staffed between the hours of 10:00 AM and 8:30 PM by two nurse practitioners and a non-TRN. The TH question was applied toward all adult patients triaged in designated triage rooms between the hours of 10:00 AM and 8:30 PM during each PDSA cycle.

Participants

Participants were limited to the accessible population of ED health care personnel within the ED at the time the project was conducted and applicable patient charts that met the inclusion criteria and were accessible for this project. TRNs were selected based solely on availability and agreement to participate. Nurses were not excluded based on years of practice or experience in triage. This project included only patient triage encounters completed in designated triage rooms. According to the hospital's current policies, all patients aged 21 years and younger should be treated within the pediatric ED. Therefore, EHR audits were only conducted on patients 22 years and older. Patient encounters and triage notes completed between FT hours, 10:00 AM and 8:30 PM, were included in this project.

Patient encounters outside of this time frame were not included. Convenience sampling was used to enlist three TRNs, two nurse practitioners, and two attending physicians for stakeholder interviews.

In summary, inclusion criteria for this project were (1) patient encounters for patients aged 22 years and older, (2) triage interviews conducted by TRNs within designated triage rooms, (3) patient encounters between the hours of 10:00 AM and 8:30 PM, and (4) stakeholder willingness to participate in interviews.

Data Collection

Approval from the institutional review board of the College of Nursing at The University of Arizona and all permissions from the hospital were obtained before beginning this QI project. Patient consent for the electronic health information exchange is obtained during registration for treatment and was therefore ensured before accessing patient EHRs. Quantitative data were obtained through EHR audits before, during, and after the TH question was implemented. Interviews with stakeholders were recorded, transcribed, and grouped into common categories according to the methods of discourse analysis.[19] Recordings were deleted once transcription was complete, and no personal identifiers were included in transcriptions.

Data Analysis

The statistical analysis software SPSS (IBM Corp, Armonk, NY) was used for data analysis in this QI project. Each category of data considered for inclusion in this project was evaluated for abnormal distributions, and outliers were excluded. The author was unable to further analyze relationships between multiple variables because of low nursing compliance with asking the TH question. The author believes it is difficult to draw definitive conclusions regarding the cause of changes to data categories included in this project because the TH question was asked so infrequently. Transcriptions of interviews were reduced and organized into a category scheme to be more manageable for grouping.[19]

RESULTS

Data are categorized into three 2-week time blocks for data comparison. Each time block, or phase, consists of 14 days total. **Table 1** illustrates the dates of importance for this project, separated into preimplementation, PDSA C1, and PDSA C2. C1 was not completed as a continuous 2-week cycle because of unforeseen circumstances. Original data were extracted by and were received from the ED Business Intelligence officer, who routinely conducts chart audits within the ED. After all exclusion criteria were applied, the total number of patient encounters included for analysis in this project were n = 841 (preimplementation), n = 838 (C1), and n = 956 (C2).

Table 1 Project phases and dates			
	Phase	**Beginning**	**End**
Date	Preimplementation	July 4, 2017	July 17, 2017
	C1	July 18, 2017	July 19, 2017
	C1, continued	July 27, 2017	August 7, 2017
	C2	August 8, 2017	August 21, 2017

This table includes the exact dates of each phase of this QI project.

Triage and Patient Placement

Extreme outliers were excluded from all time-related triage categories. Total triage times did not change or increase during the PDSA cycles when compared with preimplementation times. The mean triage time during preimplementation (n = 824) was 2.79 ± 1.88 minutes. The mean triage time during C1 (n = 812) and C2 (n = 929) were 2.29 ± 1.80 minutes and 2.66 ± 2.12 minutes, as seen in **Table 2**.

A higher percentage of patients were treated in FT after implementing the TH question. FT treated 21.52% (n = 181) of total included patient encounters during the preimplementation phase. This percentage increased during C1 to 31.62% (n = 265) and during C2 to 28.66% (n = 274). The mean ESI score for FT patients did not change across the phases. **Table 3** includes further information regarding ESI scores for FT patients. There was an overall decrease in the percentage of FT patients required to transfer to the main ED. Before implementation, 7.73% of FT patients (n = 14) were moved to an ED treatment room after being initially placed in FT. This percentage did not initially change during C1 because 7.17% of FT patients (n = 19) were moved to an ED room, and then decreased during C2 because 5.11% of FT patients (n = 14) were moved. FT length of stay decreased from an average of 172 ± 126 minutes (preimplementation) to 166 ± 104 minutes during Cycle 2. The percentage of patients admitted from FT initially decreased during C1 when compared with preimplementation, but then returned to baseline rates during C2. Of the patients initially placed into FT, 3.87% (n = 7) were admitted during preimplementation, 0.75% (n = 2) were admitted during C1, and 3.28% (n = 9) were admitted during Cycle 2.

Targeted History and Triage Notes

The TH question was asked for 26.25% of included patient encounters (n = 220) during C1 and 17.57% of included patient encounters (n = 168) during C2. For those patients asked the TH question, more than 59% (C1) and more than 65% (C2) reported a pertinent PMH related to their chief complaint (**Table 4**).

EHR chart audits revealed few triage notes specifically stated the TH question. To address this issue the author deemed it appropriate to additionally audit triage notes for information related to PMH, keeping in line with the main objectives of this project. The PMH category (see **Table 4**) was created to account for triage notes that did not state any acceptable forms of TH (previously described), but included the words "history," "past medical history," or "diagnosed." In triage notes that did not specifically state an acceptable form of TH, PMH was addressed in 31.6% (Cycle 1) and 27.2% (Cycle 2) of remaining notes.

Table 2 Triage times					
		Phase	Total, n	Mean, min	Median, min
Results	Preimplementation		824	2.79 ± 1.88	3.00
	Cycle 1		812	2.29 ± 1.80	2.00
	Cycle 2		929	2.66 ± 2.12	2.00

This tables includes information regarding the mean and median triage times for all patient encounters, which met all inclusion/exclusion criteria previously listed, included in this project.

Table 3
Fast track times

	Categories	Preimplementation	Cycle 1	Cycle 2
FT total, n (%)		181 (21.52)	265 (31.62)	274 (28.66)
ESI scores, n (%)				
5		13 (7.18)	8 (3.02)	17 (6.20)
4		133 (73.48)	191 (72.08)	204 (74.45)
3		33 (18.23)	64 (24.15)	50 (18.25)
2		2 (1.10)	1 (0.38)	3 (1.09)
N/A		0 (0)	1 (0.38)	0 (0)
Moved to ED, n (%)		14 (7.73)	19 (7.17)	14 (5.11)
FT LOS, min		172.39 ± 126.92	172.04 ± 126.51	166.48 ± 104.58
Admissions, n (%)		7 (3.87)	2 (0.75)	9 (3.28)

This tables includes information regarding FT patient encounters before and during this QI project.
  Abbreviations: LOS, length of stay; N/A, patient encounters that did not have an assigned ESI score.

There were a remaining 421 triage notes (C1) and 571 triage notes (C2) that did not meet acceptable criteria to be included in the categories of TH or PMH. Almost one-fifth (C1) and almost one-fourth (C2) of these remaining triage notes addressed the patient seeking medical treatment before visiting the ED (see **Table 4**). Patients reported most commonly seeking prior treatment from a primary care provider or specialist provider, an urgent care, or another hospital. **Fig. 1** presents a visual representation of the number of triage notes that addressed PMH or prior treatment. In total, 59% of triage notes in C1 and 54% of triage notes in C2 addressed the TH question, PMH, or the patient seeking prior treatment (see **Table 4**).

Table 4
Targeted history

	Categories	Cycle 1	Cycle 2
TH question asked? n (%)			
Yes		220 (26.25)	168 (17.57)
No		617 (73.63)	786 (82.22)
N/A		1 (0.12)	2 (0.21)
If TH asked (yes): pertinent history, n (%)			
Yes		131 (59.55)	110 (65.48)
No		90 (40.91)	58 (34.52)
If TH not asked (no): PMH, n (%)		195 (31.60)	214 (27.23)
If TH nor PMH asked: prior treatment, n (%)		84 (19.95)	140 (24.52)
Total, n (%)		499 (59.55)	522 (54.60)

This tables includes information gained from EHR audits regarding patient history within the context of the triage note. "n" for each category signifies the number of triage notes that fell into that specific category. "Total" refers to all notes that mentioned either TH, PMH, or prior treatment.

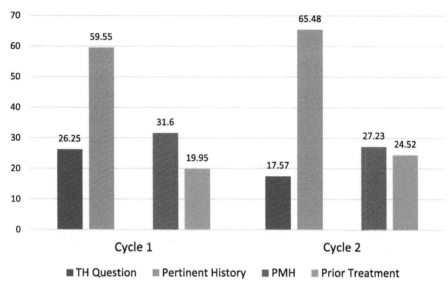

■ TH Question ■ Pertinent History ■ PMH ■ Prior Treatment

Fig. 1. TH, PMH, or prior treatment information obtained from triage note audits. This figure lists the frequency of triage notes that assessed for TH, and the number of those encounters that had a pertinent medical history related to the chief complaint. Additionally, the frequency of triage notes that addressed PMH or prior treatment (but not TH) are included.

Nursing Compliance

There were 48 triage nurses that met inclusion criteria during C1 and C2, and whose triage notes were included for data analysis. TRN compliance varied greatly from day to day (**Fig. 2**). Compliance was measured according to how many triage notes addressed TH or an accepted version of TH. The highest daily compliance was 52%, whereas the lowest daily compliance was 0% (see **Fig. 2**). Overall compliance for Cycle 1 was 25.70 ± 19% and 17.65 ± 13.37% for Cycle 2.

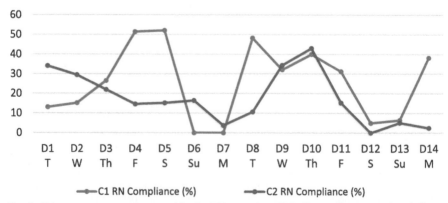

●— C1 RN Compliance (%)   ●— C2 RN Compliance (%)

Fig. 2. Triage nurse compliance with the TH question. This figure illustrates the daily RN compliance percentage, with the days numbered and correlated with the day of the week.

Interview Outcomes

Three TRNs, two attendings, and two nurse practitioners were interviewed for this QI project (n = 7). **Table 5** provides a detailed description of stakeholder answers to questions from Appendix 2, and **Table 6** provides answers to questions from

Table 5	
Stakeholder interview common related comments	
Question	**Common Related Comments**
1. What are your personal opinions regarding the QuickLook process? Feel free to provide examples of advantages or disadvantages	QL is succinct but also limits the RN (RN1, NP2) Strongly dislike QL, preferred previous triage process (RN2) QL provides the RN with unsatisfactory information because of lack of history (RN3, NP1, NP2) Unfamiliar with details of QL (MD1, MD2)
2. How do you believe QuickLook has impacted the triage process and patient placement between fast track and the ED?	No effect on triage process or patient placement (RN1, RN2, RN3) Believes 3-min time limit too restricting because of multiple responsibilities (RN2, RN3, NP2) Sometimes read triage note, but prefer to be in the room during triage or receive verbal report from triage RN (MD1, MD2) Mostly read the triage note before seeing the patient (NP1, NP2) Some triage notes are too succinct, do not provide enough information (NP1, NP2)
3. A targeted history question is a single question about PMH, worded as: "Have you been treated for this [chief complaint] before?," and is intended to be added to the QuickLook process. How do you think this will affect ESI scoring and patient placement?	Agree with or have a positive opinion of the TH question (RN1, RN2, RN3, MD1, NP1) Important to ask about PMH in triage (RN1, NP1, NP2) Sometimes, RN already asks patient about PMH during triage (RN1, RN2, RN3) Exits the QL narrator to look up patient history (RN3) The TH question will help RNs make better triage and patient placement decisions (RN3, MD2, NP1, NP2) Unaware that QL does not include PMH (MD1, MD2)
4. How feasible is it to add the TH question to QuickLook and still complete the triage interview according to Banner standards of <3 min?	Cannot identify issues with adding TH question to QL (RN1, RN3, MD1, MD2, NP2) Very feasible (RN2, NP1) Predicting maintaining <3 min standard (RN1, RN2, RN3)
5. What have you noticed about the integration of the TH question into QuickLook?	Useful information gained when TH question asked (RN1, MD1, MD2, NP1) Forgot to ask TH question (RN1, RN3) RN already asks about PMH during triage (RN2) PMH information gained during triage, before asking TH question (RN2, RN3) Low RN compliance with asking TH question (MD2, NP1, NP2) TH question relevant for determining patient placement (NP1) Desire for higher compliance with asking TH question (NP2)

This table contains answers obtained from stakeholder interviews that have been analyzed and summarized according to common themes.

Table 6
Evaluation questions: stakeholder interview common related comments

Question	Common Related Comments
6. Compared with QuickLook before the TH question, to now, how do you believe the TH question has impacted the triage process and patient placement between fast track and the ED?	Information gained from TH question was useful for determining ESI acuity (RN1, RN2, RN3) No change to triage process (RN2, RN3) Able to make more informed decision about patient placement (RN1, RN3) Information from TH question was sometimes helpful with patient placement (MD1) Answers to TH question helped place patients appropriately into FT (MD2, NP1, NP2)
7. What difficulties did you encounter with integrating the TH question into the triage process?	Unsure how to use question, at first (RN1) Unsure when to ask TH question during triage interview (RN1, RN2, RN3) Forgot to ask TH question during high patient volume times (RN1, RN2) Difficult to change routine (RN2, RN3) TH question not appropriate for chief complaint (RN2, RN3, NP2) Not involved in integrating TH question (MD1, MD2, NP1, NP2) Did not observe any difficulties with integration (MD1, MD2, NP1) Observed low RN compliance (NP2)
8. In what ways did the TH question help you with assigning an ESI acuity score and placing a patient in either fast track or the ED?	Helped in assigning acuity for chronic patient complaints (RN1, NP2) Described specific instances where RN was able to use information gained from the TH question to determine patient placement appropriate for FT (RN1, RN2) Helped identify a high-acuity patient (RN2) Asked about history before implementation (RN3) Did not ask TH (MD1, MD2, NP1, NP2) Observed that useful information obtained from asking TH question when reviewing triage notes (NP1)
9. What would you like to see changed?	The wording of the question (RN1) The TH question included in the EHR QuickLook narrator (RN2, NP1) Would like to visualize patient's history, but not ask about full PMH (RN3) PMH added to QL narrator (RN2, RN3, MD1, MD2, NP1, NP2) More education for nurses to ask PMH during triage (MD2)

This table contains answers obtained from stakeholder interviews that have been analyzed and summarized according to common themes.

Appendix 3. Stakeholders who participated in preimplementation interviews were also asked evaluation questions once the project was complete.

The following information pertains to data collected during the preimplementation phase from questions 1 to 4, listed originally in Appendix 2. Overall, stakeholders had negative feelings regarding QL, and most stakeholders mentioned the role of PMH in triage or had a positive opinion of the TH question (see **Table 5**). For question 1, almost half of stakeholders verbalized that QL did not provide the TRN with enough information during triage, because of the exclusion of PMH. For question 2, all nurses interviewed (n = 3) stated they believed QL did not have an impact on the triage process. Three out of seven stakeholders stated they believed the 3-minute time limit for QL was too restricting because of the multiple responsibilities of a triage nurse (see **Table 5**). For question 3, almost all stakeholders verbalized a positive opinion of the TH question after the TH question was explained to them. Additionally, all RNs stated they believe they already ask about PMH during some triage interviews, whereas one nurse went on to described exiting the QL narrator during triage to look up the patient's history elsewhere in the EHR. The interviewed stakeholders could not identify any issue with the prospect of implementing the TH question, or thought implementation would be feasible when asked question 4 (see **Table 5**).

Question 5 was asked during implementation, between the course of C1 and C2. More than half of stakeholders interviewed stated they believed useful information was gained when the TH question was asked (see **Table 5**). Two-thirds of TRN stakeholders stated PMH information was obtained without asking the TH question, and they forgot to ask the TH question during some triage interviews (see **Table 5**). Almost all attendings and nurse practitioners interviewed commented on the low TRN compliance rate during implementation.

The following information pertains to evaluation questions (6–9) that were asked at the end of C2. Overall, stakeholders had positive opinions associated with using the TH question (see **Table 6**). Although stakeholders encountered several issues with implementation, they reported gaining useful information when the TH question was asked (see **Table 6**). For question 6, all three nurses recounted specific situations where information was gained after asking the TH question, and this information was useful in determining an ESI score. Almost every stakeholder commented on how information gained from the TH question was useful in determining patient placement (see **Table 6**). Question 7 revealed stakeholders encountered several difficulties when implementing the TH question. Nurses were unclear on when to ask the TH question and how to integrate it into the triage interview. Interviewed nurses also found it difficult to change their "routine" during QL and reported easily forgetting to ask the TH question during times of high patient volumes (see **Table 6**). When asked what they would like to see changed (question 9), almost every stakeholder verbalized wanting PMH to be included in the QL narrator in the EHR. Stakeholders also suggested changing the wording of the TH question, integrating the question into the EHR, and providing more education to TRNs (see **Table 6**).

Summary

The primary purpose of this QI project was to integrate a TH question into QL to increase effective patient-to-nurse communication in the ED. Secondary purposes for this QI project were to identify any significant impact the TH question may have on ESI scores, patient placement, and the triage interview process.

The primary purpose of this project was achieved. TRNs were educated to integrate the TH question into the triage process. Data analysis shows that TRNs successfully integrated the TH question into triage, despite low RN compliance, and stakeholder responses show positive outcomes to asking the TH question. Quantifying the success of integration is based on data showing triage times did not change between pre-implementation and postimplementation. Secondary purposes to identify any impact on ESI scores and patient placement were partially achieved. There were several limitations to this QI project that hindered multivariate analysis, but stakeholders believed the TH question had an overall positive impact on patient placement and the triage process.

DISCUSSION

Data obtained for this QI project show triage nurses are capable of asking patients about pertinent PMH without prolonging total triage times. **Table 1** demonstrates integration of the TH question into the triage interview did not affect mean triage times when compared with preimplementation triage times. The percentage of FT patient encounters increased for C1 and C2, and there was a decline in the percentage of FT patients that needed to be moved from FT to an ED room during these cycles (see **Table 2**). The percentage of admissions from FT decreased during C1, but then increased during C2 to be equivalent to the preimplementation phase percentage of admissions (see **Table 2**). Additionally, the total length of stay for FT patients decreased during C2. As previously described, the author is limited in making any further multivariate conclusions regarding the direct effects of the TH question on these FT variables.

Although the TH question was infrequently asked, chart audits showed TRNs actively assess patients' pertinent PMH. This was demonstrated by the overall high percentage of total triage notes that mentioned a form of TH, PMH, or prior treatment (see **Fig. 1**). Nursing compliance, measured by the frequency of triage notes that addressed the TH question, was low for C1 and C2 (see **Table 3**). This is attributed to the many difficulties TRNs faced during implementation, including but not limited to: confusion surrounding the TH question, the perception of being "too busy" during high patient volumes, and forgetfulness (see **Table 4**). Almost two-thirds of patients who were asked the TH question had a history related to their chief complaint (see **Table 3**). In total, more than half of triage notes from patient encounters during C1 and C2 addressed either the TH question, PMH or a previous diagnosis, or the patient seeking prior treatment (see **Table 3**).

A significant amount of information was gained from stakeholder perceptions. Responses show nurses believed the TH question provided them with useful information for determining ESI scores and patient placement. Overall, stakeholders identified the importance of PMH in triage, had positive opinions regarding the TH question, and expressed a desire for PMH to be included in QL (see **Table 4**).

Recommendations

Based on the results of this QI project, a patient's PMH should be added to the QL narrator in the EHR program for the nurse to visualize during the triage interview. The author acknowledges unknown costs associated with altering an existing EHR program, but argues the potential to improve patient health outcomes greatly outweighs one-time monetary costs. The author does not believe asking patients for a full PMH during triage would provide any additional benefit to the TRN, but recommends all TRNs be educated on the importance of PMH in the triage decision-making process. The author recommends adding a synopsis of the patient's history into the QL narrator for the TRN to review for pertinent history, following the principle of the TH question. This allows the nurse to view patient history without needing to discuss the entirety of it with the patient.

Strengths and Limitations

There were several strengths to this QI project. The original timeframe for this project was doubled (increased from one PDSA cycle to two cycles) based on recommendations from multiple nurse practitioners and attending physicians. The timeline of this project was doubled with the intention of increasing TRN buy-in and the total number of patient encounters to be used for analysis. Trending data show that prolonging the PDSA cycles past a month would not change measured outcomes. The author was employed as a nurse in the ED during this project, but bias is excluded from compliance rates because the author did not complete any triage notes during implementation. The author did not directly participate in the triage process and did not have direct influence on what was written in triage notes. Additionally, TRNs were provided with daily reminders and visual reminders located directly next to triage computers to prompt increased compliance.

This QI project encountered several limitations. TRN buy-in and compliance cannot be excluded from bias because the author has worked as a peer with each TRN, ranging from several months to several years. The author cannot exclude that this familiarity with nurses may have impacted compliance rates with asking the TH question. The rate at which PMH or prior treatment was mentioned in triage notes was not assessed for patient encounters before the start of C1. Therefore, no comparison is made between PDSA cycles and preimplementation regarding the rate of change in which TRN asked about PMH during the triage interview. This QI project was also limited by the involvement of a single author to execute in-services. It was difficult for the author to provide a daily in-service to every TRN because the ED frequently rotates nurses throughout the day. This may have contributed to poor compliance rates. This was a single-center project conducted at an urban hospital in Southern Arizona. Results are not generalizable in QI projects. Additionally, bias cannot be excluded from the analysis of stakeholder interviews, because qualitative analysis is inherently subjective.

REFERENCES

1. Rui P, Kang K, Albert M. National hospital ambulatory medical care survey: 2013 emergency department summary tables. CDC; 2013.
2. Quattrini V, Swan BA. Evaluating care in ED fast tracks. J Emerg Nurs 2011;37(1): 40–6.
3. Kim SW, Horwood C, Li JY, et al. Impact of the emergency department streaming decision on patients' outcomes. Intern Med J 2015;45(12):1241–7.
4. Huffman KC. Increasing effective patient-triage nurse communication using a targeted history question [DNP project]. Tucson (AZ): University of Arizona; 2017.
5. Aksel G, Bildik F, Demircan A, et al. Effects of fast-track in a university emergency department through the National Emergency Department Overcrowding Study. J Pak Med Assoc 2014;64(7):791–7.
6. Emergency Severity Index [ESI]. Welcome to the emergency severity index (ESI). 2016. Available at: http://www.esitriage.org. Accessed July 1, 2016.
7. Hwang CE, Lipman GS, Kane M. Effect of an emergency department fast track on Press-Ganey patient satisfaction scores. West J Emerg Med 2015;16(1):34–8.
8. Arslanian-Engoren C. Explicating nurses' cardiac triage decisions. J Cardiovasc Nurs 2009;24(1):50–7, 8p.
9. Bansal E, Dhawan R, Wagman B, et al. Importance of hospital entry: walk-in STEMI and primary percutaneous coronary intervention. West J Emerg Med 2014;15(1):81–7.
10. Castner J. Emergency department triage: what data are nurses collecting? J Emerg Nurs 2011;37(4):417–22.

11. Ryan K, Greenslade J, Dalton E, et al. Factors associated with triage assignment of emergency department patients ultimately diagnosed with acute myocardial infarction. Aust Crit Care 2016;29(1):23–6.

12. Wolf L. Does your staff really "get" initial patient assessment? Assessing competency in triage using simulated patient encounters. J Emerg Nurs 2010;36(4): 370–4, 5p.

13. Atzema CL, Austin PC, Tu JV, et al. Emergency department triage of acute myocardial infarction patients and the effect on outcomes. Ann Emerg Med 2009;53(6):736–45.

14. Hitchcock M, Gillespie B, Crilly J, et al. Triage: an investigation of the process and potential vulnerabilities. J Adv Nurs 2014;70(7):1532–41, 10p.

15. Wolf L. Acuity assignation: an ethnographic exploration of clinical decision making by emergency nurses at initial patient presentation. Adv Emerg Nurs J 2010; 32(3):234–46.

16. Rouen P. Aligning design, method, and evaluation with the clinical question. In: Moran K, Burson R, Conrad D, editors. The doctor of nursing practice scholarly project. Burlington (MA): Jones & Bartlett Learning; 2017. p. 347–73.

17. Rouen P. Aligning design, method, and evaluation with the clinical question. In: Moran K, Burson R, Conrad D, editors. The doctor of nursing practice scholarly project. Burlington (MA): Jones & Bartlett Learning; 2014. p. 331–46.

18. Institute for Healthcare and Improvement [IHI]. Plan-do-study-act (PDSA) worksheet. 2017. Available at: http://www.ihi.org/resources/Pages/Tools/PlanDoStudyActWorksheet.aspx. Accessed May 1, 2017.

19. Polit DF, Beck CT. Nursing research: generating and assessing evidence for nursing practice. 9th edition. Philadelphia: Wolters Kluwer Health, Lippincott Williams & Wilkins; 2012.

APPENDIX 1: LITERATURE REVIEW SUMMARY

Reference	Research Question/Aims	Study Design	Sample and Setting	Methods and Data Collection	Findings
Arslanian-Engoren,[8] 2009	Explicate the decision-making processes of ED triage nurses for MI patients	Qualitative: descriptive	Setting: United States, ED Sample: 12 ED RNs (11 women, 1 man) 3 focus group sessions Age range: 25–62 y old, average 47 y old	Focus groups to help determine best approach for instrument development that can be used to quantify the decision-making process in ED triage Script used to interview ED RNs, experienced with triage Focus groups were audiotaped, recordings transcribed, data extrapolated from transcripts Themes developed from transcripts, data coded into categories	Themes in determining underlying causes patient's chief complaint: PMH, patient demographics, clinical presentation, attitudes and perceptions, cultural beliefs, nursing knowledge and experience Important patient cues: general appearance, transportation mode, cardiac history, vital signs, chest pain Determine relevant cues/triage status: life-threatening symptoms, PMH, ED staff
Atzema et al,[13] 2009	Examine triage acuity of MI patients, identify any delays to care Identify how many MI patients were triaged as low-acuity	Quantitative: retrospective cohort	Setting: Ontario, Canada, ED Sample: n = 102 acute care Canadian hospitals	Data obtained from EHR auditing	Half of AMI patients were given a low acuity triage score when they presented Independently associated with substantial delays in electrocardiogram acquisition and to reperfusion therapy Quality of ED triage important factor limiting performance on key measures of quality of AMI care

(continued on next page)

(continued)

Reference	Research Question/Aims	Study Design	Sample and Setting	Methods and Data Collection	Findings
Castner,[10] 2011	Questions: What data do triage RNs believe they are required to obtain? What data do they believe is most important? What amount of time do they believe is required to triage a patient?	Qualitative: questionnaire, descriptive cross-sectional	Setting: mailed survey, United States Sample: n = 430 returned surveys	Created list of data points on questionnaire, each including 5-point Likert scale ranging from "never," to "strongly agree" to "strongly disagree" Mailed survey to ED triage RNs registered through Emergency Nursing Association Data analysis on survey responses	429/430 respondents rated medical history as "strongly agree" when asked if they believe this is important to include in triage Other data pointed rated as "strongly agree": vital signs, allergies, pain, surgical history, weight, maltreatment scale Respondents report average time of triage was 9.03 min with standard deviation of 7.25 min
Hitchcock et al,[14] 2014	Explore and describe triage, to identify potential problems and vulnerabilities that impact triage	Qualitative: observational, ethnographic	Setting: Pre-ED, Australia Sample: 60 triage interviews 31 informal interviews 14 formal interviews 170 h of observation	In-field observations of triage and interviews with ED staff including RN. shift leaders, medical officers, clerical staff Researcher collected data while observing triage process Methods: observer only, field notes, informal and formal interviews Data = interview transcripts, field notes, diagrams, journal entries, transcripts Themes derived from information collected	Themes identifying problems/vulnerabilities in triage: "Negotiating patient flow and care delivery through the ED" "Interdisciplinary team communicating and collaborating to provide appropriate and safe care to patients" "Varying levels of competence of the triage nurse" Selected categories: triaging the patient, extended time to triage and further assessment, inexperienced triage RNs, limited triage education, triage errors

Ryan et al,[11] 2016	Identify factors associated with triage acuity in AMI patients; patient demographics, clinical characteristics, nursing triage experience in years	Quantitative: retrospective cohort	Setting: ED, Australia Sample: n = 153 AMI patients in ED	EHR charts reviewed of patients discharged with diagnosis of AMI, between June 2009 and May 2010	20% of patients undertriaged 18% of category 1 and 2 patients had cardiac history (22 out of 123 total) 30 patients with AMI undertriaged to groups 3–5 93% of undertriaged group presented with atypical symptoms (did not present with chest pain)
Wolf,[15] 2010	Explore RN understanding of patient acuity levels during triage interview, explore decision making processes, understand critical cues that determine acuity and placement	Qualitative: ethnographic	Setting: ED, two hospitals, United States Sample: n = 12 ED RN (10 triage RN, 2 nontriage RN) 120 patients 2 hospitals	Nonparticipant observation of RN and patient interaction during triage interview over 3-mo time period Simultaneous data collection and data analysis Field observations and conversations recorded via notes Analyzed for themes	RN understood acuity to be based on: patient presentation, complaint, duration of symptoms, body habitus Acuity influences by patient volume, unit leadership, communication with patients and providers, and length of time in triage Physiologic data not rigorously collected nor primary determinant of acuity Duration of symptoms influential on acuity: long and very short = less acute score Acuity perception of ESI 2 complaints influenced by duration of symptoms, age, and history of patient

(continued on next page)

(*continued*)

Reference	Research Question/Aims	Study Design	Sample and Setting	Methods and Data Collection	Findings
Wolf,[12] 2010	To identify triage nurse deficiencies in knowledge base, ability to identify critical cues, ability to ask right questions to make informed decision	Mixed methods Qualitative: ethnographic Quantitative: pretest/ posttest	Setting: ED, United States Sample: n = 40 ED RN	Developed 16 (2 pairs of 8) clinical scenarios to simulate different triage situations, with purpose of assessing whether RN able to use appropriate questions in triage RNs chose 2 numbers between 1 and 8, randomly picking their own clinical scenarios RN educator acted as simulated patient, answering triage RNs questions Second part: written test assessing acuity assignment RN educator listened to simulated triage scenarios, accompanied by checklist to determine if RN pass/fail	Only one RN correctly answered all questions on written test and passed both simulations 20% of RNs scored 10–11 points out of 13 total ESI accuracy of 48%–69% for 80% of ED staff Inaccuracy resulted from: not asking for vital signs, not have sense of working diagnosis, not taking medical history into account, ignoring out of range vitals RNs did not rely on physiologic data to make decisions RN questioning guided by triage form, not by patient statements

Abbreviations: AMI, acute myocardial infarction; MI, myocardial infarction; RN, registered nurse.

APPENDIX 2: STAKEHOLDER QUESTIONS

Before intervention:

1. What are your personal opinions regarding the QuickLook process? Feel free to provide examples of advantages or disadvantages.
2. How do you believe QuickLook has impacted the triage process and patient placement between fast track and the ED?
3. A TH question is a single question about PMH, worded as: "Have you been treated for [chief complain] before?," and is intended to be added to the QuickLook process. How do you think this will affect ESI scoring and patient placement?
4. How feasible is it to add the TH question to QuickLook and still complete the triage interview according to Banner standards of less than 3 minutes?

During intervention:

5. What have you noticed about the integration of the TH question into QuickLook?

APPENDIX 3: EVALUATION QUESTIONS

1. Compared with QuickLook before the TH question, to now, how do you believe the TH question has impacted the triage process and patient placement between fast track and the ED?
2. What difficulties did you encounter with integrating the TH question into the triage process?
3. In what ways did the targeted TH question help you with assigning an ESI acuity score and placing a patient in either fast track or the ED?
4. What would you like to see changed?

The Application of the Toyota Production System LEAN 5S Methodology in the Operating Room Setting

Treasa 'Susie' Leming-Lee, DNP, MSN, RN[a],*,
Shea Polancich, PhD, RN[b], Bonnie Pilon, PhD, RN-BC, NEA[c]

KEYWORDS

- Quality improvement • Lean • Operating room • 5S • Distractions • Interruptions
- Toyota Production System • Waste

KEY POINTS

- OR distractions and interruptions potentially interfere with surgical workflow contributing to patient safety risks and increase care provider stress leading to types of medical errors.
- The TPS Lean methodology identifies eight wastes, (1) defects, (2) over-production, (3) waiting, (4) confusion, (5) motion, (6) excess inventory, (7) over processing, and (8) human potential.
- The TPS 5S tool process is a space organizing process and consist of the following five elements: sort, straighten, shine, standardize, and sustain.
- The application of the TPS's Lean 5S tool process in the OR can lead to elimination of process waste related to distractions and interruptions creating a safe and efficient patient care delivery environment.
- The specific aim of the TPS 5S Lean QI project was to evaluate the impact of the TPS 5S tool process on distractions and interruptions in the neurosurgery OR workflow with a goal to decrease neurosurgery craniotomy infection rates from 9.0 per 100 cases to 4.4. per 100 cases (2010 national benchmark) in a neurosurgery OR suite within a 3-month period.

Disclosure Statement: There are no relationships with a commercial company that has a direct financial interest in the subject matter or materials discussed in article or with a company making a competing product.
[a] Vanderbilt University School of Nursing, 461 21st Avenue South, 216 Godchaux Hall, Nashville, TN 37240, USA; [b] Clinical Innovation for Quality Improvement, UAB Nursing Partnership, UAB School of Nursing and UAB Hospital, University of Alabama, Birmingham, Birmingham, AL MEB 314B, USA; [c] Vanderbilt University School of Nursing, Vanderbilt University, 461 21st Avenue South, 220 Godchaux Hall, Nashville, TN 37240, USA
* Corresponding author.
E-mail address: Susie.leming-lee@vanderbilt.edu

Nurs Clin N Am 54 (2019) 53–79
https://doi.org/10.1016/j.cnur.2018.10.008
0029-6465/19/© 2018 Elsevier Inc. All rights reserved.

INTRODUCTION

The Institute of Medicine's (IOM) report, "To Err is Human: Building a Safer Health Care System" indicated "that at least 44,000 Americans die each year as a result of medical errors" and the "total national costs ... of preventable adverse events ... are estimated to be between $17 billion and $29 billion, of which health care costs represent over half."[1(pp1–2)] A comprehensive approach was recommended by the IOM to address the complex problems to build a safer health system. As a follow-up to the "To Err is Human: Building a Safer Health Care System," the IOM published the report, "Crossing the Quality Chasm: A New Health System for the 21st Century." This report provided a framework for redesigning the American health care delivery system for the twenty-first century. The committee recommended 6 aims or dimensions that quality should exhibit: safety, effectiveness, patient-centered, timeliness, efficiency, and un-biased or equitable.[2]

It is estimated that 40% to 50% of hospital medical errors take place in the oper-ating room (OR).[3] Surgical site infections (SSIs) are one type of these medical errors. This type of infection occurs in more than 500,000 patients annually.[4] SSIs contribute to an increased length of stay, a reduced quality of life, and death.[5] On average, 2.7% of surgeries result in SSIs.[6] From a cost perspective, SSIs are thought to account for up to $7 billion annually in health care expenditures.[7] Hawn and colleagues[8] estimate that 40% to 60% of SSIs are preventable.

Distractions and interruptions are frequent contributing factors to medical errors. In the OR, these contributing factors are especially prone to result in errors, such as SSI, an adverse event stemming from an error, that impacts patient outcomes.[9] The pur-pose of this article is to present the story, from a previously unpublished quality improvement (QI) Lean 5S methodology project, of how SSIs were reduced as a by-product or outcome of removing distractions and interruptions in the surgical workflow of a neurosurgery OR through the application of the Toyota Production System (TPS) 5S, a simple, but powerful QI tool.

Problem Description

The problem observed in the neurosurgery OR by the neurosurgical team was distrac-tions and interruptions occurring in the surgical workflow due to unnecessary foot traffic related to the OR neurosurgical team searching for supplies, medications, and medical equipment. The organization's staff and surgical team satisfaction survey contained one question related to distractions and interruptions, *necessary materials and equipment are available when I need to perform my job*, which showed a rating of 0.0725, a significantly low score, which supported the observed problem. The organi-zation's safety survey was also reviewed. Using a scale of fail, poor, acceptable, very good, and excellent, only 61% of respondents indicated the *overall patient safety as very good or excellent.*

The unnecessary foot traffic, a distraction and interruption in the surgical workflow, in this neurosurgery OR was confirmed through a Lean spaghetti diagramming exer-cise (**Fig. 1**). "A spaghetti diagramming is a visual representation using a continuous flow line tracing the path of an item or activity through a process. The continuous flow line enables process teams to identify redundancies in the workflow and oppor-tunities to expedite process flow."[10(p1)] Such opportunities include identifying methods to shorten the walking time from one activity to another for frequently per-formed tasks. Another benefit of the visual drawing is to highlight major intersection points within the logistical setting. Areas where many walk paths overlaps are causes of delay one of the 8 wastes of Lean, as is unnecessary motion.[10]

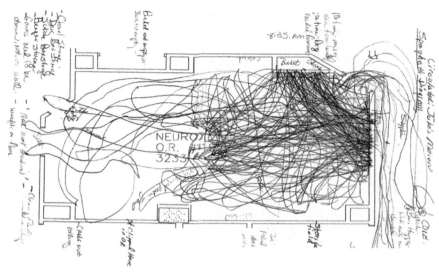

Fig. 1. Spaghetti diagram of neurosurgery OR foot traffic.

After completing the neurosurgery OR spaghetti diagramming exercise, multiple loops in the foot traffic patterns were identified as well as overlaps. These traffic patterns identified multiple back-and-forth motions to obtain supplies and equipment due to the placement of these items in the OR; crossing the surgical field to obtain supplies and equipment; and making multiple exits out of the OR in search for supplies, equipment, and medications leading to the opening and closing of the OR doors. These distractions and interruptions were thought to be a possible cause for an increase in neurosurgery SSIs, 9.0 per 100 cases, a decrease in staff satisfaction with availability of supplies and equipment, and an increase in cost because of overstocking of neurosurgical surgical supplies because staff did not trust the supplies would be readily available when needed.

Available Knowledge

OR distractions and interruptions potentially interfere with surgical flow, contribute to patient safety risks, and increase care provider stress, leading to medical errors.[3] Wheelock and colleagues[11] found in a recent study that distractions occurred in 98% of surgical cases and at a rate of 10.94 distractions per case or one distraction every 10 minutes. The most frequent types of distraction were those initiated by external staff entering the OR. The study also found that such distractions were unnecessary in 81% of cases.[11] Although the study attributed less significance to the major outcome variables (such as teamwork or stress), it was acknowledged as the potential impact on surgical infection rates, which they did not monitor.

"Controlling the OR environment to maintain proper air flow is a worldwide issue."[12(p668)] Excessive foot traffic in and out of the OR can lead to airflow disruption and airborne contamination that may increase the risk of SSIs and can cause distractions that can lead to errors.[13] It has been previously established that increased crowding in the OR is associated with a higher postoperative infection rate.[14,15] Door openings disturb the engineered airflow of the OR, which can seed the air above the incision with bacteria from the patient's skin, the operative staff, and areas outside the OR.[13]

Wheelock and colleagues[11] also measured intensity of distractions. They found that the most intense distractions were those that were equipment related (eg, wrong or missing equipment). Equipment-related distractions impacted all aspects of teamwork and stress levels for nurses. Such distractions occurred about once every 90 minutes. These medical errors contribute to the development of complications in more than half of reported complications, and the rate may be even higher. The review of medical errors that result in harm often focuses on human error; however, the actual occurrence of medical errors is often more complex. "Factors related to the specific systems, processes, and personnel all contribute to the occurrence from medical error, but systems issues are involved in 90% of errors resulting in adverse events."[3(p546)]

ORs are also resource intense and costly. "Most surgical dollars are spent in the OR, making it a high-priority target for efficiency efforts."[14(p371)] Maximizing OR efficiency becomes critical to maintaining an economically viable institution.[4] Efforts to increase OR efficiency need to be counterbalanced against the impact on patient and staff satisfaction, and more importantly, the impact on patient and staff safety, and finally, the impact on patient clinical outcomes.[4] Because of the widespread increase in OR foot traffic, The Joint Commission, as part of its SSI Change Project, promoted a reduction in OR foot traffic as an effective practice to reduce SSIs.[15]

A variety of improvement methodologies have been proposed as a partial solution to address these health care inefficiencies, such as the waste in the system, the growth in health care costs, and patient safety. The TPS Model, an automotive-based improvement Lean methodology, was created by the world-class automaker, Toyota, and is now being adapted as a means to reduce health care inefficiencies and improve safety.[16]

Rationale

The TPS Model (Lean methodology) emerged in manufacturing in the United States around 1992 and in the health care arena in the early 2000s.[16] It is a rigorous improvement system designed to transform waste, excess inventory, waiting/delays, overproduction, unnecessary transporting, unnecessary motion, defects/mistakes, excess possessing, and confusion,[17] into value from the customer's perspective.[18] This improvement methodology approach is best represented as a house with 2 pillars: those pillars are Respect for People and Continuous Improvement. The foundation of these 2 pillars has 5 elements: challenge, kazien (continuous improvement), genchi genbutus (go and see), respect, and teamwork.[19] The Respect for People pillar addresses growing leaders who understand the work, developing exceptional people and teams that follow the organization's philosophy, and respecting the suppliers by challenging them and helping them to improve.[19] The Continuous Improvement Pillar offers 5 stages of improvement, which include (1) value to the customer, created by the producer and defined in terms of specific products with specific capability offered at specific prices; (2) value stream mapping, which identifies the end-to-end process; (3) flow, which stipulates that products move smoothly and directly from process to process without waiting or waste; (4) customer pull, which creates a new production dynamic away from batches and queues; and (5) perfection, the reminder that TPS methodology embraces a continuous improvement mentality[16] and attempts to remove nonvalue activity, simplify processes, and satisfy the customer delivery needs.[20] The tactical knowledge that underlies the TPM methodology is captured in 4 basic rules: "Rule 1, all work shall be highly specified as to content, sequence, timing, and outcome; Rule 2, every customer-supplier connection must be direct, and there must be an unambiguous yes-or-no way to send requests and receive responses; Rule 3, the pathway for every product and service must be simple and direct; and Rule 4, any improvement must be in accordance with the scientific method, under the guidance of a teacher, the lowest possible level in the organization."[21(p98)]

Lean 5S tool process

TPS provides several tools to reduce waste in the system, but one tool, 5S, encourages streamlined inventories, clutter-free workspaces, and processes to maintain housekeeping standards. The TPS 5S (**Fig. 2**)[22] is a scientific process that "identifies visually the standard and deviations from the standard through standardization of work practices implemented to reduce distractions and interruptions in the surgical flow process by standardizing everyday work practices."[19(p161)] This tool is being used in health care to reduce inventory, create space, and reduce travel and search times. Graban[23] states that little attention has been given to the effects of 5S on safety; however, several have suggested that safety is an important aspect of 5S tool methodology.[16]

Each stage of a TPS 5S Project has an impact on safety and efficiency, from the *sorting* function, whereby broken or expired items are removed, to sustain, whereby ongoing cleaning, maintenance, and standard of work checks are routinely conducted. In the first step, sort (*Seiri*), removing expired or broken items from the work areas, can increase safety by decreasing the chance of using improper items for patient care. An effective visual method to identify these unnecessary items is called *red tagging*. A red tag is placed on all items not required to complete the job.[16,24] In the straighten or set in order (*Seiton*), step 2, frequently used items will be easily accessible, improving ergonomics. Set in order or straighten focuses on efficient and effective storage and workplace organization methods and can be summarized with the adage, *A place for everything and everything in its place.*[16,24] The third step, shine (*Seiso*), ensures that all items, areas, and equipment are clean and properly maintained, which prevents

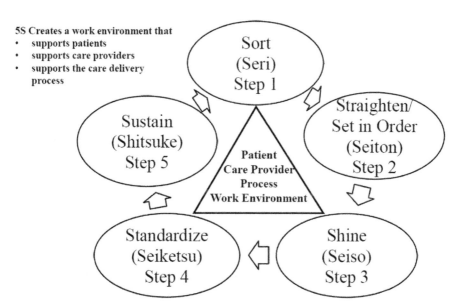

Fig. 2. The TPS 5S process tool. (*Adapted from* 5S Creating a Visual Healthcare Workplace Cycle-Diagram, Jimmerson, 2014; and *Data from* Jimmerson C. Review: realizing exceptional value in everyday work. 3rd edition. Bozeman (MT): CareOregon Inc; 2014.)

contamination and equipment being out of service. One of the main benefits of the shine step is that workers develop a sense of pride and ownership in a clean and organized work area.[16,24] Standardize (*Seiketsu*), the fourth step, improves safety by allowing all providers to quickly assess when items are unfit for use, not in their proper place, or not properly cleaned or maintained. Standardization also allows providers to find items quickly.[16,24] Employees are often a valuable source of information for the development of these standards. The fifth step, sustain (*Shitsuke*), creates mechanisms for maintaining the first four S's over time.[16,24] Many organizations find themselves returning to *doing things the same old way* only a few months after a 5S project. One key practice to prevent this return to old habits is routine observation of the standard work practices and checking to ensure that the 5S discipline is being followed.[25]

Understanding that surgery is a high-risk activity,[26,27] "it would naturally be expected that there would be a high level of control in the operating theatre environment, a high level of reliability in equipment and a low level of control of interference overall."[27(p603)] However, studies show that there is a high level of distractions and interruptions in surgical flow processes that have the potential to increase the occurrence of surgical errors, such as incorrect counts, retained foreign bodies, wrong medications, wrong site surgery,[26] and SSIs (waste) related to unnecessary OR foot traffic and searching for supplies and equipment needed for the surgical case.[13] If the application of the TPS's 5S tool process is adapted in the OR, the waste related to distractions and interruptions may be eliminated and variation decreased, creating a safe, efficient, and effective health care delivery workflow system.

Specific Project Aim

The specific aim of the QI project is to evaluate the impact of the TPS 5S tool process on distractions and interruptions in the neurosurgery OR workflow with a goal to decrease neurosurgery craniotomy infection rates from 9.0 per 100 cases to 4.4. per 100 cases (2010 national benchmark) in a neurosurgery OR suite within a 3-month period. **Table 1** list project goals and objectives that support this aim to decrease work process distractions and interruptions.

METHODS

This QI project applied the TPS 5S tool process design for eliminating distractions and interruptions in the neurosurgery OR suite workflow to prevent craniotomy SSIs. The TPS's 8 forms of waste were the platform for the project providing direction needed to meet the aim of the project. The TPS 5S tool consists of organizing space in accordance with the specific steps of *sort*, necessary items from unnecessary items; *straighten*, organize and label the location for items; *shine*, clean the workplace, and equipment is cleaned and prepared for use; *standardize*, develop cleaning methods and cleanliness standards to maintain first 3Ss; and *sustain*, review the workplace regularly, making it a habit.[16] The TPS 5S tool principles provided the knowledge to carry out the project. The TPS's Lean 5S project work was accomplished through the use of the systematic, scientific Plan, Do, Study, and Act (PDSA) cycle of change model (**Fig. 3**),[28] an iterative, 4-phase model used for improving a process or carrying out change, "emphasizing the role of learning in improvement".[29(p331)]

Context

The OR leadership team and the TPS 5S Project Team decided that there was a need to conduct an assessment to gather baseline data before implementing a change. The

Table 1

Toyota Production System 5S project goals, outcomes objectives, and tactics for the functional domain

Goals	Outcomes Objectives	Action Tactics
Goal 1: Equipment: To provide a structured approach and easy to understand methodology for OR organization, order, and cleanliness for equipment by August 2010	1. 90% of the surgical team will agree or strongly agree that all required equipment for the surgical case is in the OR by February 2011 2. 90% of surgical team will agree or strongly agree that all required equipment is in working order by February 2011 3. 90% of the surgical team will agree or strongly agree that all required equipment in the OR is clean by February 2011 4. 90% of the surgical team will agree or strongly agree that all equipment in the OR has a designated location by February 2011	To provide a method for ensuring clean, working, equipment, to include instruments, are available for each the surgical case by: 1. Establishing a surgical team to focus on application of the 5S process: Sort, Straighten, Shine, Standardize, and Sustain by August 2010 2. Creating a Sort Inspection Sheet for items not essential to the OR (items not touched in 3 mo should be removed from the area) by August 2010 3. Identifying items in the OR not necessary in the area and red tag the items by August 2010 4. Locating the red tag items to a staging area by July 2010 5. Determining disposition of the red tagged items by August 2010 6. Establishing standards for basic organization and orderliness by August 2010 7. Creating a 5S cleaning plan for the area and determine the evaluation period by September 2010

(continued on next page)

Table 1
(continued)

Goals	Outcomes Objectives	Action Tactics
Goal 2: Supplies: To provide a structured approach and easy to understand methodology for OR organization, order, and cleanliness for supplies by September 2010	1. 90% of the surgical team will agree or strongly agree that all required supplies for the surgical case are in the OR by February 2011 2. 90% of the surgical team will agree or strongly agree that all required medications, including blood, needed for the surgical case are in the OR by February 2011	To provide a structured approach for ensuring supplies, to include medications and blood, are available for each the surgical case by: 1. Establishing a cross-functional team to oversee improving the supply process; the team will include: supply chain coordinator, OR director, manager of OR pharmacy, circulator nurse, OR manager, OR administrator by August 2010 2. Flow charting the supply and equipment process to remove non-value-added steps by August 2010 3. Establishing and implementing standards for basic supply organization and orderliness by August 2010 4. Creating Sort Inspection Sheet for supply items not essential to the area (if an item has not been touched in 3 mo it should be removed from the area) by August 2010 5. Identifying items that are not necessary in the OR area and red tag the items by August 2010 6. Locating red tagged items to a staging area by August 2010 7. Determining disposition of the red tagged items by November 2010

Goal 3: Space: To create and implement a visual management system and organized physical OR space to improve workflow by August 2010	1. 90% of the surgical team will agree or strongly agree that multiple items in the OR are grouped and placed in the same location by February 2011
	2. 90% of the surgical team will agree or strongly agree that storage areas in OR are clearly labeled by February 2011
	3. 90% of the surgical team will agree or strongly agree that the physical layout of the OR allows for equipment and supplies to be easily accessed by November 2010
	4. 90% of the surgical team will agree or strongly agree that the physical layout of the OR allows for patient information to be easily accessed by February 2011
		To create and implement a visual management system that will ensure adherence to standards of work reducing confusion, reduce errors, encourage staff involvement, and reduce stress by:
		1. Providing just-in-time training, "providing job training coincidental with or, immediately before, an employee's assignment to a new or expanded job"[17(p606)], for visual management and space organization to the OR care providers by August 2010
		2. Identifying standards for the visual management system in the OR by August 2010
		3. Creating a visual display and standards to be posted by August 2010 (see **Fig. 11**)
		4. Creating and implementing a visual management implementation plan by August 2010
		  a. Designating target areas with a timeline for training and implementation
		  b. Selecting a 5S champion for target OR area
		  c. Creating a Visual Management Worksheet
		  d. Standardizing OR visual management system

Goal 4: OR foot traffic: To create and implement a visual management system to organize the OR space to prevent unnecessary OR foot traffic by August 2010	1. 90% of the surgical team will agree or strongly agree that OR foot traffic has decreased by February 2011	To develop and implement an OR Foot Traffic policy to stabilize new foot traffic practice that includes how to communicate the need for equipment, supplies, medications, and similar when they are not available in the OR 1. Only required surgical team members are present in the OR during the surgical case 2. Surgical team members leave the OR during the surgical case only for breaks and lunch 3. When the surgical team does not have the equipment or supplies needed to start a case, there is a clear process for communication of such problems to resolve them in a timely manner 4. When the surgical team does not have the equipment or supplies needed to start a case, there is a clear process for communicating such problems to resolve them in a timely manner

- Adopt the change or
- Abandon the change or
- Run through the cycle again, possibly under different conditions, different materials, different people or different rules –Deming

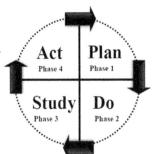

- State objectives of the test of change
- State scope of the PDSA
- Make predictions, surfaces the theory, experience, hunches, world views
- Develop a plan to carry out test of change
- Develop a data collect plan

- Complete the analysis of the data
- Compare data to predictions
- Summarize what was learned

- Carry out test of change
- Document problems and unexpected observations
- Begin analysis of the data

Rapid Cycles of Change

Fig. 3. PDSA is an iterative, 4-phase problem-solving model used for Improving a process or carrying out change. (*Adapted from* Langley GJ, Nolan KM, Nolan TW, et al. The improvement guide: a practical approach to enhancing organizational performance. 1st edition. San Francisco (CA): Jossey-Bass Publishers; 1996; with permission.)

assessment consisted of a review of the current literature regarding the types of distractions and interruptions that affect the surgical team's performance and review of the previous OR safety surveys. The literature search showed that instruments, supplies, room logistics, communication, and operating foot room traffic were the items that lead to the most significant distractions and interruptions.[8] After discussion with the stakeholders, the OR leadership team and the TPS 5S Project Facility Group, it was decided that the current data did not provide the information needed to determine the needs of the neurosurgery surgical team. The OR leadership approved administering a baseline Neurosurgery OR Functional Needs Assessment Survey and the Neurosurgery Surgical Team Satisfaction Survey to gather perceived needs of the surgical team focusing on distractions and interruptions in the ORs.

The Neurosurgery OR Functional Needs Assessment survey questions were developed based on a literature search and a human factor's expert's knowledge. Equipment, supplies, motion, visual signals, and logistics were the major categories for questions. The Neurosurgery OR Functional Needs Assessment Survey and the Neurosurgery Surgical Team Satisfaction Survey were distributed electronically through the organization's e-mail system. The surveys' convenience sample (n = 131) was drawn from a population of 582 surgeons, nurses, anesthesiologists, certified nurse anesthetists, and surgical technologists. The surveys' respondents ranged from aged 25 years to greater than 55 years.

Based on the Neurosurgery OR Functional Needs Assessment Survey results, with all responses less than 90% (**Table 2**), and with a score of 90% on Neurosurgery Surgical Team Satisfaction Survey question responses deemed of significance by the OR stakeholders, the OR Leadership concluded that the organization was not providing the surgical team with the tools needed to perform safe, timely, efficient, effective, and patient-centered care in the OR. Leadership acknowledged a need to move forward with the implementation of the TPS 5S Project to meet the needs of the surgical team by reducing distractions and interruptions. Forces to support this action plan included the results of the needs assessment survey, and the perceived needs were very powerful in providing a valid description of the situation[30]; regulatory requirements to create a safe patient care environment; and a need to improve surgical

Table 2
Preneurosurgery operating room functional needs assessment results

Neurosurgery OR Functional Needs Assessment Survey Questions	Disagree or Strongly Disagree (%)	Agree or Strongly Agree (%)
Equipment		
1. All required equipment being used for the surgical case is in the OR	83.3	16.7
2. All required equipment in the OR is in working order	66.7	20
3. All required equipment in the OR is clean	63.4	33.3
4. All required equipment in the OR has a designated location	66.6	13.3
Supplies		
5. All required supplies for the surgical case are in the OR	86.6	3.3
6. All supplies in the OR are visible and in the open	76.6	13.3
7. All medications, including blood, needed for the surgical case are available in the OR	40.0	33.3
Visual signals and organization of physical space (logistics)		
8. Multiple items in the OR are grouped and placed in the same location	73.4	10.0
9. Storage areas in the OR are clearly labeled	60	23.3
10. The physical layout of the OR allows for equipment and supplies to be easily accessed	30.0	56.7
11. The physical layout of the OR allows for patient information to be easily accessed	66.7	16.7
OR foot traffic		
12. Only required surgical team members are present in the OR during the surgical case	53.3	33.3
13. Surgical team members leave the OR during the surgical case only for breaks and lunch	50.0	36.6
14. When the surgical team does not have the equipment or supplies needed to start a case, there is a clear process for communicating such problems to resolve them in a timely manner	63.3	20.0
15. When the surgical team does not have the equipment or supplies needed to start a case, there is a clear process for communicating such problems to resolve them in a timely manner	31.34	42
16–19. Questions are demographics in the body of the article		

team satisfaction. A barrier to the plan was the surgical team's lack of knowledge of the 5S system, but the OR leadership viewed the 5S tool process training of the surgical team as the remedy for this opposing force.

Setting

This project took place in a neurosurgery OR at a large urban, academic, tertiary acute care hospital in the southeastern United States. The operative services department consists of more than 800 employees, 83 ORs which includes 6 neurosurgery ORs in 7 primary procedural locations, 3 free-standing ambulatory surgery centers in the community, and performs more than 50,000 procedures annually.

The project team included the chair of the neurosurgery department, one neurosurgeon, 2 anesthesiologists, one nurse anesthetist, one anesthesia technologist, one plant services staff member, one housekeeping staff member, one neurosurgery OR manager, 2 neurosurgery OR nurses, the director of perioperative QI, and the perioperative QI project manager. All participants were selected because they were closest to the OR work, which is critical to the success of a QI project.

Intervention/Change

This project was implemented over a 12-week period. The PDSA cycle of change was used to guide implementation of the intervention/change. Each phase included key steps in the process.

Plan phase

The following steps were taken to begin the TPS 5S project:

1. Met with the OR leadership team to gain approval of the 5S Lean project.
2. Selected the distractions and interruptions in the OR workflow as the process for improvement with the OR leadership.
3. Selected the specific OR where the project would be implemented.
4. Recruited a multidisciplinary TPS 5S Project Team.
5. Developed a TPS 5S project action plan and data collection plan.
6. Distributed preimplementation the Neurosurgery OR Functional Needs Assessment Survey.
7. Contacted the organization's infection control department and the perioperative informatics department to gain approval to obtain needed project data.
8. Met with the TPS 5S neurosurgical team to determine project prediction, project goals, and objectives.
9. Photographed the selected neurosurgery OR before 5S implementation.
10. Created plan to provide just-in-time 5S training for the TPS 5S Team.

Do phase

The following steps were taken to implement the TPS 5S tool in the neurosurgery OR:

1. Conducted a 2-hour 5S tool process just-in-time training session, which included presenting a 5S tool video specific to health care. Instructions were provided on how to proceed in conducting the 5S tool process by the TPS 5S lead along with distributing the neurosurgery OR floor plan for mapping the new organization of the OR.
2. The TPS 5S Project Team then conducted the 5S event just after the training, where all TPS 5S Project team members met in the OR and began the 5S process. The TPS 5S Project Team began by first *sorting* all items located in the OR, which included red tagging all unnecessary items and removing them from the OR. This was followed by the *straighten step*, organizing the neurosurgery OR according to the OR surgical team requirements and 5S principles using the OR floor plan to strategically draw with a pencil (for this publication the drawing is in an electronic format) where all equipment and supplies where to be placed in the OR (**Fig. 4**). Then came the *shine step*: the OR was cleaned, equipment and electrical cords were rearranged or placed in a safer location to improve access to OR supply doors and to provide a straight and safe pathway from the OR hall door to the center of the OR where the OR table is located. The anesthesia machine was also repositioned to allow for clearer walk pathway.

   Issues discovered during the 5S event day related to the *shine step*, which could not be accomplished during the 1-day event, were addressed later. These

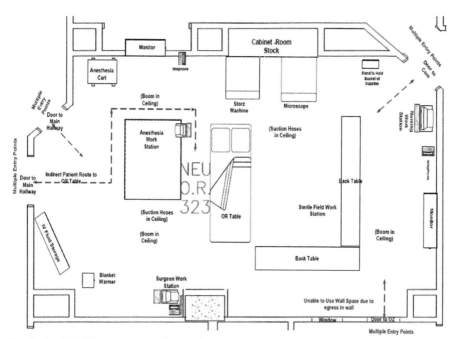

Fig. 4. Pre-TPS 5S Lean Project physical layout of neurosurgery OR.

challenges included installation of a new, larger hallway OR door, with a new automatic door opener, to allow ease of entry into the OR for the patient and staff; extra exit doors and observation windows in the OR were removed from the wall to increase wall space. Because of the relocation of the surgical table, the lights were rearranged, and the entire OR was painted. After these issues were resolved, the OR was given one last *shine* due to the construction. The *standardize step* followed. During this step, all needed equipment and supply locations were replaced in the OR, color-coded, and labeled, and plastic floor angles were used to define the floor equipment space, allowing the OR surgical team to immediately know when a piece of equipment is missing from the OR. Photographs were taken of each piece of equipment, laminated, and posted behind each piece. The OR surgical team developed *Before Start of Day and at End of Day Equipment and Supplies Checklists* that were laminated and posted in the OR. These checklists were followed during the *sustain step*, which included a daily logistic checklist that was reviewed each morning and evening by the circulating nurse or designee to ensure all needed equipment and supplies were available and in the right place. Cleaning procedures for the OR were posted and reviewed each day.

3. The 5S project lead photographed the selected neurosurgery OR after the 5S implementation to provide evidence of the OR change to the OR leadership as well as the TPS 5S Project Team.
4. An OR Foot Traffic policy was implemented to stabilize steps taken to reduce unnecessary OR foot traffic.
5. The TPS 5S Project Team lead distributed the postimplementation functional survey and neurosurgery surgical team satisfaction survey to the neurosurgery team 6 weeks after the 5S process.

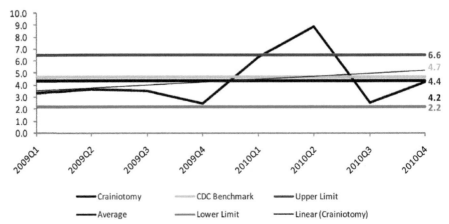

Fig. 5. Craniotomy procedure infection rates before the implementation of the 5S Lean Project and immediately after the implementation of the 5S Lean project.

Study phase of intervention/change

The Do and Study phases of the PDSA cycle were used to study 5S tool intervention/change. The TPS 5S Project Team studied the impact of the intervention/change, which began in the Do phase (this is the phase whereby analysis or the study of the intervention/change data begins), of the project by reviewing any documented problems and unexpected observations that occurred in this phase. In the Study phase of the PDSA cycle, the TPS 5S Project Team continued to study the intervention/change by using the following tools:

a. Control charts were used by the TPS Project Team to study the impact of the 5S tool process intervention/change on the craniotomy infection rates, a defect or error waste, over the project period and over a 7-year period after the project ended. An initial control chart (**Fig. 5**) was used to determine if the project aim was met over a 3-month period. Two x-control charts were used to study of impact of the intervention/change over the 7-year period to determine the sustainability of the intervention/change (**Figs. 6** and **7**). The TPS Project Team used the initial control to evaluate the clinical outcome of re-organizing the OR space and providing the needed surgical case equipment and

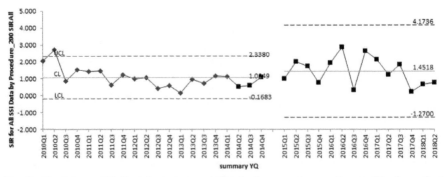

Fig. 6. Craniotomy SIR that includes superficial, deep, and organ/space SSIs from first quarter 2010 to second quarter 2018.

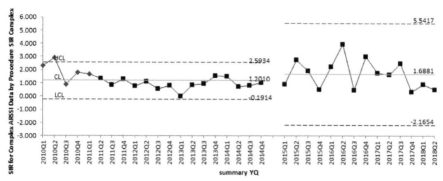

Fig. 7. Craniotomy SIR for complex ARSSID between first quarter 2010 and second quarter 2018 that only include deep incisional primary SSIs organ/space SSIs. CL, control limit; CDC, Centers for Disease Control and Prevention; LCL, lower control limit; UCL, upper control limit; YQ, Year/Quarter.

supplies in the OR suite to reduce unnecessary foot traffic, a process waste of motion.

b. A run chart was used to study the impact of the 5S tool process intervention/ change on the cost reduction of the neurosurgery inventory biplane carts. The TPS Project Team monitored the run chart over time to determine the effectiveness of placing needed supplies directly in the OR suite instead of using the supplies located on the biplane carts outside of the OR suite. These biplane carts were over-stocked due to the OR team's belief that the supplies would not be readily available in the OR suite (**Fig. 8**).

c. A pre- and post-Neurosurgery OR Functional Needs Assessment survey was used to study the neurosurgery's OR team's perceptions of the neurosurgery OR functional work processes. The data from these surveys were placed in a comparative data table. The TPS Project Team used this comparative data to evaluate the 5S

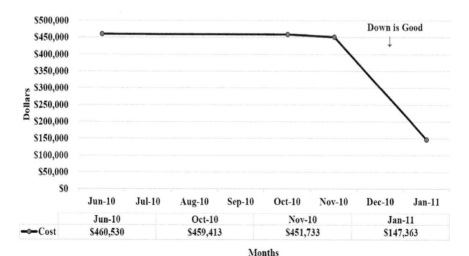

	Jun-10	Oct-10	Nov-10	Jan-11
Cost	$460,530	$459,413	$451,733	$147,363

Months

Fig. 8. Neurosurgery inventory reduction: waste eliminated and cost reduced by placing needed supplies in the neurosurgery OR suite and removing excessive inventory, waste, from the biplane carts.

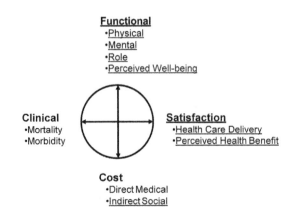

Fig. 9. The clinical value compass used to evaluate the effectiveness and efficiency of the TPS 5S Lean Project. (*From* Langley GJ, Nolan KM, Nolan TW, et al. The improvement guide: a practical approach to enhancing organizational performance. 1st edition. San Francisco (CA): Jossey-Bass Publishers; 1996; and *Reprinted from* Practice-Based Learning and Improvement: a Clinical Improvement Action Guide. Oakbrook Terrace (IL): Joint Commission on Accreditation of Healthcare Organizations; 2012. p. 83; with permission. © Joint Commission Resources.)

tool process intervention/change's impact on the neurosurgery OR functional work processes.

d. A pre- (baseline) and post-Neurosurgery Surgical Team Satisfaction Survey were used to study the neurosurgery surgical team's satisfaction with the OR workflow process. Data from these surveys were placed in a comparative data table, and the TPS Project Team used these data to evaluate the 5S tool process intervention/change's impact on the neurosurgery OR team's work satisfaction.

Act phase

The Act phase of the PDSA is whereby the OR leadership team makes the decision to either adopt the change, adapt the change, or abandon the change. This phase of the PDSA is addressed in the Discussion section of this article.

Measures

The Clinical Value Compass Model (**Fig. 9**)[28] was used to evaluate the effectiveness and efficiency of the TPS Lean 5S Project's measures. The Clinical Value Compass Model represents 4 essential measurement domains. Those domains consist of 4 cardinal points: (1) *clinical*, which includes mortality, morbidity, complications; (2) *functional*, which includes perceived well-being and work process status; (3) *satisfaction*, which includes patient, surgical team satisfaction with the work environment, and stakeholders; and (4) *costs*, which includes direct and indirect cost.[31] The Clinical Value Compass and the PDSA model are highly suited for the evaluation of clinical setting improvement projects because both models allow for a balanced and meaningful profile of caregiving processes and outcomes.[31] For this project, measures occurred in all 4 domains. In the clinical domain, the neurosurgery craniotomy infection rates were measured; in the functional domains, the availability of equipment and supplies, medications, the visual signals and organization of physical space (logistics), and the OR foot traffic was measured. In the satisfaction domain, the OR staff satisfaction was measured, and in the cost domain, the reduction in cost of neurosurgery OR biplane (supply) carts were measured.

Analysis

Descriptive and inferential statistical analysis has been used to carry out this project. Quantitative data after assessment survey results were analyzed from electronic surveys, an OR electronic database, the organization's informatics system, and electronic safety reports. Comparative analysis, using a *t* test, was conducted between the presurvey and the postsurvey data collected in the value compass domains functional and satisfaction. The *t* test was selected based on the analysis of 2 separate groups with known variances that were assumed to be equal. The level of statistical significance was set at an alpha of 0.05. Statistical process control was used to analyze the primary process measure of craniotomy infection rates, the clinical domain, displayed on x-control charts showing the evolution of the intervention/change over time. The rules for differentiating special versus common cause variation for the control charts were applied. A run chart was used to track improvements in the value compass cost domain.

Ethical Considerations

After successfully presenting the TPS 5S Lean Project proposal to the 5S Lean Project's committee chairpersons, the TPS 5S Lean Project application was submitted to the organization's institutional review board (IRB) as a QI initiative. The IRB approved the TPS 5S Lean Project, and the project was implemented. Because this was a QI project, no informed consent was required.

RESULTS
Clinical Domain

Results of the data from pre-TPS 5S Project implementation to the post-TPS 5S Project implementation indicate that there was a significant decrease in craniotomy infection, and this decrease met the project aim. Although the first 2 quarters' rates rose sharply, by the third quarter there was an infection rate of 2.6 infections per 100 procedures, which was below the national benchmark and considerably lower than the previous quarter (see **Fig. 5**). This decrease occurred after the implementation of the TPS 5S Project. Although there is a slightly upward trend, an overall rate for the 4th quarter shows the data is still within the upper limit of 6.9 and the lower limit of 1.7 infections per 100 procedures. To determine if the decrease in the craniotomy infection rates was sustainable over time, a request was made to the infection control department for the infection rate data ranging from the first quarter of 2010 to the second quarter of 2018. The Craniotomy Standardized Infection Ratios (SIR) All SSI Data by Procedure moving range control chart, that reflects surgical site infection types that includes superficial, deep, and organ/space SSIs, from 1st quarter 2010 to 2nd quarter 2018 indicates (see **Fig. 6**) there had been a sustained improvement of the craniotomy infection ratios over time, there was only common cause variation in the process, no special causes were observed. The SIR for complex/admission/readmission surgical site infection deep (ARSSI) data procedure moving range control chart, first 2010 and second quarter 2018, that only includes deep incisional primary SSIs organ/space SSIs, indicates (see **Fig. 7**) that there is a sustained improvement of the craniotomy infection ratios overtime, again the only common cause in the process, and no special cause was observed.

The infection control department informed the project lead that in 2015 the neurosurgical craniotomy SSIs' risk factors baseline changed from trauma, bed size (of the hospital, such as large >500 beds or small hospital), age at time of surgery, and duration of surgery to trauma, American Society of Anesthesiologists score, age,

Table 3
t Test: 2-sample assuming equal variances: neurosurgery before and after needs functional domain survey

	Variable 1	Variable 2
Mean	23.07857143	47.45
Variance	200.8371978	210.7303846
Observations	14	14
Pooled variance	205.7837912	—
Hypothesized mean difference	0	—
Df	26	—
t Stat	−4.494945442	—
P (T ≤ t) one-tail	6.37444E−05	—
t Critical one-tail	1.705617901	—
P (T ≤ t) 2-tail	0.000127489	—
t Critical 2-tail	2.055529418	—

procedure duration, body mass index, and wound class. The re-baseline period is higher, but still the fluctuation of the points within the control limits results from common variation inherent in the process.

Functional Domain

Results of the neurosurgery OR functional needs survey subset, with the percent of satisfied or dissatisfied, are presented in **Table 3**. Analysis of the 14 questions, using the scale of disagree/strongly or agree/strongly agree and neither agree or disagree, revealed areas of needs being met or not met in the workplace to support desired outcomes. General findings for the 5 categories of concern are synthesized in the following discussion.

The findings of the neurosurgical team need analysis in **Table 3** shows −4.49494 ($P > .05$), and the degrees of freedom (*df*) 26 indicate that there was a statistical difference in the surgical team's needs being met before the implementation of the TPS 5S Project and after the implementation of the TPS 5S Project. **Figs. 4** and **10** represent the OR space reorganization before and after the TPS 5S Project.

To determine if the TPS 5S Project goals were met, the agree and strongly agree categories for the before and after question responses were compared, and a *t* test was conducted on each survey question to determine statistical significance in the work areas before and after the implementation of the TPS 5S process. Seven of the 14 question responses showed a statistical significance. **Table 4** shows each question's response percent in the equipment, visual signals and organization of physical space (logistics), and OR foot traffic categories increased, but did not meet the TPS 5S Project outcome objective of 90%. The supply category showed an increase, but the increase was minor compared with the other question responses. Although all question responses showed a percentage increase, only 7 of the question responses showed a statistical significance.

Satisfaction Domain Results

The results of the neurosurgical team satisfaction survey subset with percent of satisfied or very satisfied are presented in **Table 5**. Analysis of the 6 questions using the scale of satisfied/very satisfied revealed areas of individual satisfaction and team

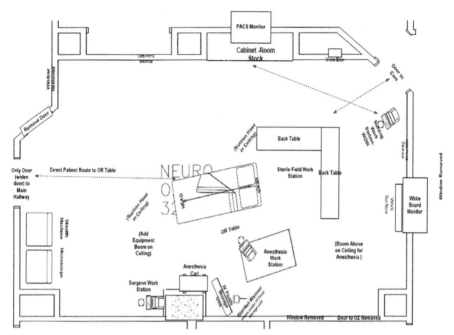

Fig. 10. Post-TPS 5S Lean Project physical layout of neurosurgery OR. PACS, picture archiving and communication system.

satisfaction with the work environment and the implication of workflow processes to support desired outcomes. General findings for the 6 survey questions of concern are synthesized in the following discussion.

A comparative analysis using an independent measures *t* test was conducted to analyze the satisfaction data collected before the TPS 5S Project and upon completion of the TPS 5S Project. The *t* test was selected based on the analysis of 2 separate groups with known variances that were assumed to be equal. The level of statistical significance was set at an alpha of 0.05.

The independent measures *t* test (**Table 6**) shows 0.992387368 (*P*>.05) and the *df* 10, indicating there is no statistical difference in the neurosurgical team's satisfaction before the implementation of the TPS 5S Project process and upon completion of the TPS Lean 5S process. To determine if the TPS 5S Project objectives were met in the satisfied and very satisfied categories, the before and after question responses were compared, and a *t* test was conducted on each survey question (see **Table 6**) to determine statistical significance with satisfaction in the workplace preimplementation and postimplementation of the TPS 5S Project. Only 1 out of the 6 questions exceeded the 90% metrics meeting the TPS 5S Project outcome objective. The *t* test performed on each question showed no statistical difference in the preimplementation and postimplementation of the TPS 5S Project.

Cost Domain

The results of the cost domain indicator, the neurosurgery inventory reduction, were tracked manually over time using a run chart. The neurosurgery inventory reduction measure results (see **Fig. 8**) show a significant decrease in inventory cost from $460,530.00 to $147,363.62, a savings of $313,166.38, and a 68% reduction in inventory. This reduction not only was a cost savings but also allowed for the eliminating of 2

Table 4
t test: 2-sample assuming equal variances: neurosurgery before and after needs functional survey for each survey question

		Neurosurgery Operating Room Functional Needs Survey: Before and After Results			
	Questions	Pre-Lean 5S Agree/Strongly Agree (%)	Post-Lean 5S Agree/ Strongly Agree (%)	T Stat	P (T ≤ t) 2 tail
	Equipment				
Question 1.	All required equipment being used for the surgical case is in the OR	10	32 (↑)	−2.5261	0.014441618
Question 2.	All required equipment in the OR is in working order	20	42.8 (↑)	−2.7034	0.009114038
Question 3.	All required equipment in the OR is clean	33.3	46.4 (↑)	−1.8604	0.068185312
Question 4.	All required equipment in the OR has a designated location	13.3	57.1 (↑)	−3.799	0.000365176
	Supplies				
Question 5.	All required supplies for the surgical case are in the OR	3.3	21.4 (↑)	−1.8613	0.068044459
Question 6.	All supplies in the OR are visible and in the open	13.3	42.9 (↑)	−3.142	0.002702013
Question 7.	Multiple items in the OR are grouped and placed in the same location	33.3	75 (↑)	−3.9963	0.000193124
	Visual signals and organization of physical space (logistics)				
Question 8.	Storage areas in the OR are clearly labeled	10	60.7 (↑)	−4.8243	1.15391E-05
Question 9.	The physical layout of the OR allows for equipment and supplies to be easily accessed	23.3	35.7 (↑)	−1.2909	0.202150252
Question 10.	The physical layout of the OR allows for patient information to be easily accessed	56.7	67.9 (↑)	−1.3088	0.196058972
Question 11.	All medications, including blood, needed for the surgical case are available in the OR	16.7	42.9 (↑)	−3.65	0.000584807
	OR foot traffic				
Question 12.	Only required surgical team members are present in the OR during the surgical case	33.3	57.1 (↑)	−1.8558	0.068850124
Question 13.	Surgical team members leave the OR during the surgical case only for breaks and lunch	36.6	39.3 (↑)	−0.4046	0.687368665
Question 14.	When the surgical team does not have the equipment or supplies needed to start a case, there is a clear process for communicating such problems to resolve them promptly	20	42.9 (↑)	−3.0782	0.003245

Table 5
Neurosurgery team satisfaction survey: before and after results

| | Questions Pre-lean 5S Post-lean 5S | | | |
	Satisfied/ Very Satisfied	Satisfied/ Very Satisfied	T Stat	P (T ≤ t) 2 tail
Question 4.	The chance to do different things from time to time	96.2	95.7 (↓)	−0.560636358	0.577708451
Question 12.	The chance to do something that makes use of my abilities	88.5	100 (↑)	−0.830954532	0.410200871
Question 16.	The freedom to use my judgment	96.2	95.7 (↓)	0.410378442	0.683393178
Question 17.	The chance to try my methods of doing the job	88.4	82.6 (↓)	0.658808387	0.513233599
Question 18.	The working conditions	88.4	83.9 (↓)	−1.228609397	0.225334824
Question 20.	The feeling of accomplishment I get from the job	96.1	95.7 (↓)	0.084058371	0.933367044

Table 6
t test: 2-sample assuming equal variances: before and after neurosurgical team satisfaction survey

	Variable 1	Variable 2
Mean	92.3	92.26666667
Variance	17.944	51.72266667
Observations	6	6
Pooled variance	34.83333333	—
Hypothesized mean difference	0	—
df	10	—
t Stat	0.00978232	—
P (T ≤ t) one-tail	0.496193684	—
t Critical one-tail	1.812461102	—
P (T ≤ t) 2-tail	0.992387368	—
t Critical 2-tail	2.228138842	

large inventory carts, which increased OR space capacity. This action was another step toward reducing the waste of excessive inventory by making supplies available to the OR surgical team at the right time and right place.

DISCUSSION

During the Act phase of the PDSA, the project results and the impact of the project are discussed with the management team to determine if the intervention/change will be adopted, abandon, or adapted. Upon review of the project results, the OR leadership team determined the project results were consistent with the literature that indicates elimination of distractions and interruptions can improve workflow in the ORs and reduce SSIs. However, because of the short implementation period of the TPS 5S Project, no conclusion could be made regarding the ultimate impact of the TPS 5S Project. The team found that there was progress toward reduction in the waste of defects (SSIs), the waste of motion (OR foot traffic due to unavailability of equipment, supplies, medications), the waste of confusion (visual signals and organization of physical space [logistics]) management as shown by the statistical positive difference in neurosurgery OR needs survey responses after the TPS 5S Project. Since the initial review of results, there is evidence of a significant positive decrease in neurosurgery craniotomy infections meeting the project aim, which has been sustained over a 7-year period. The strengths of the project were also identified by the OR leadership. One of the major strengths of the project was the support and commitment of the OR leadership and from the OR neurosurgery staff, particularly the multidisciplinary 5S team, who invested their time and expertise to develop project aim, project goal, and project objective, and to ensure work tasks were addressed. The use of a proven scientific improvement methodology, 5S, including its rules, principles, and tools along with the PDSA cycle of change, and using the value compass to evaluate the project work, were discussed as project strengths. These improvement methodologies are grounded in testing and learning cycles and provided a defined set of tools to understand the process and test the process, embraced a psychology and logic, and considered the contexts of justification and discovery.[32]

INTERPRETATION

Although all action plan goal tactic activities were completed, and the 4 overall project goals were met, the outcome objectives requiring a score of 90% or higher score on the postimplementation survey were not met. However, the staff and chief of neurosurgery did push for expansion of the project to 3 other neurosurgery OR suites, and to the neurosurgery supply room. These rooms were reorganized using the 5S tool, and antidotal comments indicated that the neurosurgery surgical team and staff are very satisfied with the new logistical arrangement of the ORs and the supply room. Over the next 6 months, the 5S tool was used to improve other services' supply rooms because of the immediate impact of the process on improving the staff's ability to find the needed supplies and equipment and reducing OR foot traffic.

LIMITATIONS

There are limitations regarding the interpretation of the TPS 5S Project data because several other practices were standardized and addressed during this project period (eg, skin preparation practices, flash sterilization, OR attire, normothermia, glycemic control, and hair removal). The project occurred in only one OR setting, the neurosurgery OR, so the results are not generalizable. The short change period was also a limitation of the TPS 5S Project, although the work has been sustained for 7 years and the SSI rates remain lower than when the project was implemented. Change over time is important to determine if a change is effective and if a change is sustainable. It cannot be stated that the trends noted were solely due to the implementation of the TPS 5S Project, which was designed as a part of a multifaceted project to prevent SSIs.

SUMMARY

The TPS 5S Project can provide a beginning platform for removing distractions and interruptions of the surgical flow processes, allowing ORs to meet their mission to improve the health status of individuals and communities served by providing safe, patient-centered, cost-effective surgical health services. These types of TPS 5S Projects can lead to improved patient clinical outcomes and reduction of excessive resources, leading to cost savings. This type of project can also improve care provider satisfaction, reducing turnover and increasing operational productivity because the OR surgical team no longer spends valuable time searching for items needed to perform their work, leading to a more satisfying work setting. The TPS Lean tools, strategies, and principles bring value to the care provider's everyday work processes. It is that scientific, experiential approach to learning that ensures sustainability of those work processes into the future.

Lessons learned, which are used to improve future projects and future stages of current projects,[33] included recognizing through data that waste, distractions, and interruptions do interfere with the workflow. If one wants to eliminate this waste, they must create new systems and processes through innovative methods, such as the use of the TPS 5S Lean tool process. It was learned that just-in-time training is an effective method to educate and train the OR surgical team, who had little to no knowledge of the Lean methodology and little time to spend in training on how to implement the 5S tool process. The authors learned the importance of posting visual management standard work tools, such as the Neurosurgery OR Standardize and Sustain Checklists (**Fig. 11**), and using color-coded vinyl floor marking angles and adding photographs of equipment posted above the equipment to ensure the team knows the exact location for each piece of equipment to act as a communication tool for people who perform the necessary work to ensure the 5S changes are sustained. One item that was very important to sustain the change was developing and implementing an OR Foot Traffic Policy to stabilize new foot traffic practice that includes how to communicate the need for equipment, supplies, medications, and so forth when they are not available in the OR. The authors also learned that the scientific, systematic PDSA cycle is critical to ensure that the Lean 5S tool meets the customer's needs (value) and gives structure to the project work tactics; that it does take a *village* to successfully implement a change, all stakeholders who are closest to the work are needed to make a change that leads to an improvement; and most importantly, the authors learned that one must go to *Gemba* (where the truth is, where the work occurs) to make the change, and "one must learn by doing the thing, for though you think you know it, you have no certainty until you try."[34(p4)] At the end of TPS 5S Project, the test of change results, the strengths of the project, the limitations of the project, and lessons learned were presented to the OR leadership. Based on these elements and the discussion of the project, the OR leadership decided to accept the TPS 5S Project test of change and spread the test of change by conducting additional PDSA cycles in the remaining 5 neurosurgery ORs and the neurosurgery supply room. **Table 7** provides lessons learned regarding barriers to the 5S project and the tactics to remove those barriers.

Achieving the highest levels of organizational performance requires a well-executed approach to organizational and personal learning that includes sharing knowledge through systematic improvement. To reduce future workflow interruptions and distractions by OR surgical team members and external staff, better organization of various work tasks and deliberate design of joint activities, communication processes,

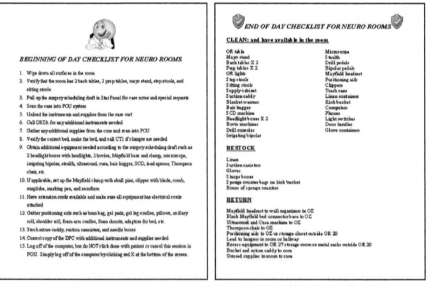

Fig. 11. Visual management tools to standardize the neurosurgery OR beginning and end-of-day work process to sustain the 5S tool interventions/changes decreasing the waste of motion/travel, defects, waiting/delays, excess inventory, confusion, and human potential. CT1, clinical technician 1; DPC, doctors preference card; ORTA, Operating room technical assistant; POU, point of use; SCD, sequential compression.

Table 7	
Lessons learned: obstacle encountered and strategies used for waste reduction	
Obstacle Encountered	**Strategies Used for Establishing a Framework and Discipline for Waste Reduction**
• Physical building layout posed obstacles to equipment installation/ placement and traffic pattern redesign	• Involve surgical team in designing layout of redesign of OR; provide floor plan showing current layout and a blank floor plan to allow team to design new layout • Actual placement of equipment and supplies in the proposed redesign locations; when you draw the redesign items, space is underestimated in a drawing • Verify and confirm final renovation cost • Add a 10% contingency cost for any budget overrun • Create a "punch list" of "to dos" after each 5S event and confirm agreement with each department involved in completing the tasks • All surgical team members sign off on floor plan/OR logistics: sign/ add signature on the floor plan document • After diagram of OR orientation for each type of procedures that are performed in the room
• Storage areas inadequate and scattered	• Define storage area proximity to related work areas: feeder linkage systems, that is, storage areas, equipment rooms, supplies areas • Develop and implement "big picture" storage system
• Lack of storage for special items (microscopes, stealths, and so forth)	• Redesign OR space for special item capacity; create new traffic pathways
• Poor maintenance of surgical equipment	• Implement preventative maintenance project; daily checklists; ownership must belong to the people doing the work
• Searching for items	• Remove unnecessary doors; clearly label of items using color coding and zoning • Implement daily *standard of work checklist* (items required in the OR at beginning of case—checked at close of cases each day and before cases begin each day)

• Negative surgical staff perceptions of the effectiveness of the TPS 5S Lean process	• Provide tangible proof of efficacy of TPS 5S Lean process; 2 approaches:
	  ○ TPS Lean 5S event
	  ○ TPS Lean 5S video most effective in showing the efficacy of TPS 5S
	• Multidepartmental approach to redesign of OR and linkage systems: clinical engineering, plant services, infection control, environmental services, pharmacy, central supply, surgical services, risk management, and finance

• Lack of resources	• Provide leadership with potential savings related to creating a clean, orderly environment where there is a place for everything and everything4 is in its place
• Cleanliness of space	• After cleaning procedures for each OR
• Technological restraints	• Investigate products and alternative processes (WOW, Nursing Documentation WorkStation On Wheels, gives logistic flexibility)

and information transfer are recommended. Although the cost of the TPS's 5S Project is relatively low, the benefits of the project are considerable in that the evaluation can inform organizational actions in ways that improve the OR conditions for both the surgical team and the patient while also meeting the organization's strategic plan and mission by creating a more effective, efficient, safe, timely, and reliable delivery of patient care.

REFERENCES

1. Kohn LT, Corrigan JM, Donaldson MS, editors. To err is human: building a safer health system. A report of the committee on quality of health care in America; Institute of medicine. Washington (DC): National Academies Press (US); 2000. Available at: https://www.ncbi.nlm.nih.gov/books/NBK225188/. Accessed September 10, 2018.
2. Briere R. Crossing the quality chasm: a new health system for the 21st century. Washington, DC: National Academy Press; 2001.
3. Marshall MB, Emerson D. Patient safety in the surgical setting. Thorac Surg Clin 2012;22(4):545–50.
4. Meeks DW, Lally KP, Carrick MM, et al. Compliance with guidelines to prevent surgical site infections: as simple as 1-2-3? Am J Surg 2011;201(1):76–8.
5. Anthony T, Murray BW, Sum-Ping JT, et al. Evaluating an evidence-based bundle for preventing surgical site infection: a randomized trial. Arch Surg 2011;146(3): 263–9.
6. Haessler S, Connelly NR, Kanter G, et al. A surgical site infection cluster: the process and outcome of an investigation—the impact of an alcohol-based surgical antisepsis product and human behavior. Anesth Analg 2010;110(4):1044–8.
7. Najjar PA, Smink DS. Prophylactic antibiotics and prevention of surgical site infections. Surg Clin North Am 2015;95(2):269–83.
8. Hawn MT, Vick CC, Richman J, et al. Surgical site infection prevention: time to move beyond the surgical care improvement program. Ann Surg 2011;254(3): 494–501.
9. Feil M. Distractions in the operating room. Pennsylvania Patient Safety Advisory 2014;11(2):45–53. Available at: http://patientsafety.pa.gov/ADVISORIES/Pages/201406_45.aspx.
10. Bialek R, Grace L, Duffy GL, & Moran JW. American Society for Quality [ASQ]. (n.d.) Spaghetti diagram. Available at: http://asq.org/learn-about-quality/process-analysis-tools/overview/spaghetti-diagram.html. Accessed September 10, 2018.
11. Wheelock A, Suliman A, Wharton R, et al. The impact of operating room distractions on stress, workload, and teamwork. Ann Surg 2015;261(6):1079–84.
12. Rovaldi CJ, King PJ. The effect of an interdisciplinary QI project to reduce OR foot traffic. AORN J 2015;101(6):666–81.
13. Lynch RJ, Englesbe MJ, Sturm L, et al. Measurement of foot traffic in the operating room: implications for infection control. Am J Med Qual 2009;24(1):45–52.
14. Fong AJ, Smith M, Langerman A. Efficiency improvements in the operating room. J Surg Res 2016;204(2):371–83.
15. The Joint Commission. (2013). Implementation guide for NPSG. 07.05. 01 on surgical site infections: The SSI change project. 2013. Available at: https://www.jointcommission.org/assets/1/18/Implementation_Guide_for_NPSG_SSI.pdf. Accessed August 25, 2018.
16. Young TP, McClean SI. A critical look at Lean thinking in healthcare. Qual Saf Health Care 2006;17(17):382–6.
17. Chalice R. Improving healthcare using Toyota Lean Production methods, 46 steps for improvement. 2nd edition. Milwaukee (WI): ASQ Quality Press; 2007.

18. Kim CS, Spahlinger DA, Kin JM, et al. Lean healthcare: What can hospitals learn from a world-class automaker? J Hosp Med 2006;1(3):191–9. Available at: https://deepblue. lib.umich.edu/bitstream/handle/2027.42/50679/68_ftp.pdf?sequence=1&isAllowed=y. Accessed November 1, 2018.
19. Liker JK, Hoseus M. Toyota culture the heart and soul of the Toyota Way. New York: McGraw Hill; 2008.
20. Nave D. How to compare Six Sigma, Lean, and the Theory of Constraint. Qual Progr 2002;35(3):73–8.
21. Spear S, Bowen HK. Decoding the DNA of the Toyota Production System. Harv Bus Rev 1999;77(5):95–106.
22. Jimmerson C. Review: realizing exceptional value in everyday work. 3rd edition. Bozeman (MT): CareOregon Inc.; 2014.
23. Graban M. Lean hospitals, Improving quality, patient safety, and employee satisfaction. New York: Productivity Press Taylor & Francis Group; 2009.
24. Ikuma LH, Nahmens I. Making safety an integral part of 5S in healthcare. Work 2014;47(2):243–51. Available at: http://web.a.ebscohost.com.proxy.library. vanderbilt.edu/ehost/pdfviewer/pdfviewer?vid=1&sid=75cdae54-d305-43aa-96fd-aac211884329%40sessionmgr4008. Accessed August 1, 2018.
25. Hill AV. 5S. 2009. Available at: http://www.clamshellbeachpress.com/downloads. php. Accessed August 19, 2013.
26. Wiegmann DA, ElBardissi AW, Dearani JA, et al. Disruptions in surgical flow and their relationship to surgical errors: an exploratory investigation. Surgery 2007; 142(5):658–65.
27. Healey AN, Sevdalis N, Vincent CA. Measuring intra-operative interference from distraction and interruption observed in the operating theatre. Ergonomics 2006; 49:589–604.
28. Langley GJ, Nolan KM, Nolan TW, et al. The improvement guide: a practical approach to enhancing organizational performance. 1st edition. San Francisco (CA): Jossey-Bass Publishers; 1996.
29. Westcott RT, editor. The certified manager of quality/organizational excellence handbook. 4th edition. Milwaukee (WI): ASQ Quality Press; 2014.
30. Kettner PM, Moroney RM, Martin LL. Designing and managing Projects and effectiveness-based approach. 3rd edition. Los Angeles (CA): Sage Publications; 2008.
31. Nelson EC, Batalden PB, Lazar JS, editors. Practice-based learning and improvement: a clinical improvement action guide. Oakbrook Terrace (IL): Joint Commission Resources, Incorporated; 2007.
32. Perla RJ, Provost LP, Parry GJ. Seven propositions of the science of improvement: exploring foundations. Qual Manag Health Care 2013;22(3):170–86.
33. Rowe SF, Sikes S. Lessons learned: taking it to the next level. Paper presented at PMI® Global Congress 2006. North America, Seattle, WA. Newtown Square (PA): Project Management Institute; 2006. Available at: https://www.pmi.org/learning/ library/lessons-learned-next-level-communicating-7991. Accessed August 19, 2018.
34. Sophocles. 5th century BCE. 2017. Available at: http://www.cambridge.org/us/ education/news/learning-not-spectator-sport/. Accessed August 16, 2018.

Implementation of a Nurse-Driven CAUTI Prevention Algorithm

Jensine A. Russell, DNP, RN[a],*,
Treasa 'Susie' Leming-Lee, DNP, MSN, RN[b], Richard Watters, PhD, RN[c]

KEYWORDS

- CAUTI • Algorithm • Evidence-based practice • Nurse empowerment
- Visual management • Model for Improvement • Leader rounding

KEY POINTS

- Catheter-associated urinary tract infections (CAUTIs) are costly but preventable hospital-acquired infections.
- The Healthcare Infection Control Practices Advisory Committee (HICPAC) recommends incorporating evidence-based clinical practice guidelines into nursing care delivery models to prevent CAUTIs.
- The implementation of an evidence-based catheter removal algorithm, visual management principles, nurse empowerment, and leader rounding was piloted to reduce an unanticipated increase in CAUTIs.
- The 6-week project using the Model for Improvement resulted in a 36% CAUTI incident rate reduction and zero CAUTIs.

INTRODUCTION

Catheter-associated urinary tract infections (CAUTIs) are costly but preventable hospital-acquired infections (HAIs) that "increase the length of stay by 2 to 4 days and cost an additional $400 to 500 million yearly in the United States."[1] These infections are associated with "unnecessary antibiotic use, [an] estimated 13,000 attributable deaths annually, and are the leading cause of secondary blood stream infections with a probable 10% mortality rate."[2] In 2008, Medicare changed the health care delivery model by charging penalties when hospitalized Medicare patients acquired

Disclosure Statement: None.
[a] Inpatient Medicine, Vanderbilt University Medical Center, Nashville, TN, USA; [b] Vanderbilt University School of Nursing, 461 21st Avenue South, 216 Godchaux Hall, Nashville, TN 37240, USA; [c] Vanderbilt University School of Nursing, 461 21st Avenue South, 220 Godchaux Hall, Nashville, TN 37240, USA
* Corresponding author. 1100 3rd Avenue North, Apartment 455, Nashville, TN 37208.
E-mail address: Jensine.russell712@gmail.com

Nurs Clin N Am 54 (2019) 81–96
https://doi.org/10.1016/j.cnur.2018.11.001
0029-6465/19/© 2018 Elsevier Inc. All rights reserved.

preventable conditions, including CAUTIs.[3] By 2009, the Healthcare Infection Control Practices Advisory Committee (HICPAC) updated the 1981 US Centers for Disease Control and Prevention (CDC) clinical guidelines for CAUTI prevention. To reduce CAUTIs, HICPAC recommended quality improvement programs, administrative infrastructure, and surveillance strategies.[4] These clinical guidelines are intended to assist health care organizations in their CAUTI prevention strategies and, by not incorporating them into their care delivery models, they are at risk for higher rates of HAIs.

BACKGROUND

In September 2016, at an urban academic medical center on the adult cardiovascular thoracic step-down unit (SDU), the CAUTI incidence rate reached a high of 14.60, compared with the target rate of 1.91. The nurse leader investigated all 4 CAUTIs diagnosed in the previous 2 months, met with the infection control nurse partner, but could not determine a common cause for the increased infections. The team reviewed the literature and discovered that the use of nursing algorithms to manage indwelling urinary catheters (IUCs) successfully decreased CAUTIs in similar clinical settings. The nurse leader developed a plan to decrease the CAUTI incidence rate that used evidence-based practice (EBP). The purpose of the project was to empower the registered nurses (RNs) to use a CAUTI prevention nurse-driven algorithm. The aim was to implement a nurse-driven, evidence-based CAUTI reduction algorithm for 6 weeks to decrease the risk of CAUTIs and reduce the CAUTI rate by 50% from 4.80 to 2.40 per 1000 catheter days.

SIGNIFICANCE

The reduction of all HAIs is significant to the health care system: shorter hospital stays, decreased use of antibiotic therapies, and $9.8 billion dollars annually, of which CAUTIs account for one-quarter of these costs.[5] In the United States, the cost for these additional days of treatment are estimated to be $424 to $451 million dollars each year for 90,000 hospital days.[6] The cost of unnecessary antibiotics add $980 to $2900 to a patient's hospitalization.[6] The projected cost of hospital-acquired CAUTIs is between $1200 and $2700 per episode.[7]

Nursing care improves when policies are based on the translation of research into clinical practice guidelines. Nurses are empowered to provide care at the highest level of their scope of practice, which improves nursing outcomes. When care is not evidence based and the need for the IUC is not consistently assessed, the risk of the patient acquiring a CAUTI increases by 5% each day the IUC remains in place.[8]

EVIDENCE-BASED PRACTICE

A relevant EBP definition is a "problem-solving approach to clinical decision making that involves the conscientious use of the best available evidence."[9] A comprehensive literature review, summarized in **Table 1**, identified effective tactics to reduce the number of CAUTI infections. The evidence-based research on CAUTI prevention indicated that the implementation of a nurse-driven algorithm was the most effective way to reduce these HAIs. Secondary successful CAUTI prevention practices included IUC assessment reminders embedded in the electronic health record (EHR)[6,7,10,11] and the use of catchphrases or mnemonics to educate nursing staff.[7,12–15] Six of the studies used the HICPAC guidelines for the basis of their CAUTI reduction strategies. Four studies showed that there was a positive impact on nurse empowerment as the result of efforts to decrease CAUTIs. All studies resulted in statistically significant

Table 1
Literature review

Reference	Methodology	Overall Findings
Timmons et al,[1] 2017	Average IUC dwell time data collected 3 mo before intervention and 3 mo after intervention Developed and implemented a nurse-driven protocol to remove IUCs Average IUC dwell time based on charge nurse data collection of IUC insertion and removal dates Retrospective chart reviews also conducted	Average IUC dwell times decreased from 4.64 d to 4.14 d Protocol not used consistently because of lack of strict monitoring Increased number of travel nurses and high staff turnover may have affected results
Oman et al,[14] 2012	Hospital-wide intervention: mandatory policy IUC insertion and care module Standardize urinary drainage products Educate ancillary staff Unit interventions included: hour education sessions; increased number of bedside commodes; purchased bladder scanner; TRIP fliers; charge RN catheter rounds; family and patient education materials regarding IUC care (English and Spanish)	Decreased IUC catheter days CAUTI rates not affected Bladder scanner was a useful tool to avoid possible IUC reinsertion Policy module made staff aware of best practices for IUCs and potential for CAUTIs Mandatory reeducation about proper IUC insertion made this skill more important Standardization of products saved the hospital $52,000 and did not result in an increased CAUTI rate
Andreessen et al,[10] 2012	Updated current procedures and protocols for catheter use, insertion, and maintenance into a bundle Mandatory staff education Standardized insertion kits containing a closed drainage system and a securement device Advocated for use of external condom catheters Purchased bladder scanners Computerized daily assessment of IUC, including elements for clinical indications and removal	Process measures: Documentation compliance: daily catheter use, 98%; new order template, 35%; insertion removal template, 40%; indication, 45% Outcome measures: Catheter device days: 71% overall (505–148 d) Reduction in use: 56% Feedback is an essential component to keeping staff involved in the process Multidisciplinary teamwork Poor timing of MD education
Marra et al,[13] 2011	Phase 1: ICU RNs and MDs inserted UCs Phase 2: bladder bundle: UC insertion cart; hand hygiene; CHG and meatal antisepsis; sterile field and gloves; 1 attempt for each attempt; adequate UC balloon inflation; daily review of need for UC with prompt removal if no longer needed Education of study protocol Encouraged participation in UC Bundle Getting to Zero program Daily ICU rounds to remove unnecessary UCs Two indications: 1. Close I&O monitoring 2. Patient requiring vasopressors Sporadic use of bladder scanners Daily CHG baths for all UC patients	UC use in ICU from 0.62 to 0.53 and 0.18–0.12 in SDU CAUTI rate decreased in ICU from 7.6 per 1000 catheter days to 5.0 and in SDU from 15.3 to 12.9 CAUTI rates were higher in SDU than ICU

(continued on next page)

Table 1
(continued)

Reference	Methodology	Overall Findings
Underwood,[15] 2015	Used Comprehensive Unit-Based Safety Program education to evaluate impact on urinary catheter use and CAUTI rates Insertion techniques Catheter care Positioning of drainage bag Appropriate urinalysis and culture testing criteria Proper documentation and prompt removal Staff signed a document to agree to implement the goals IUC indications mnemonic: HOUDINI	Reduced catheter days by 14% Reduced catheter use by 14% Reduced CAUTIs by 19% Alternative IUC devices for men only are condom catheters Nursing leadership can empower health care providers to deliver excellent patient care
Gokula et al,[7] 2012	Used IAMS instead of PDSA: I: identifying A: assessing I: implementing M: modifying/maintaining S: spreading/surveillance FIRM protocol CUCIS	Charge nurse input was valuable FIRM not used because a lot of UCs placed in OR CUCIS not used because of a lack of clear direction related to responsibility and process Simplified FIRM and CUCIS Developed nurse-driven system IUC program to be included in new RN orientation Plans to integrate orders into EHR Continued surveillance of new IUC policy Mandatory annual education
Mori,[6] 2014	Preintervention needs assessment Evaluated the effectiveness of a nurse-driven removal protocol and how it affected the incidence and duration of IUC use as well as CAUTI rates Protocol allowed nurses to discontinue IUC without MD order when indications not met Online education, poster board, one-on-one reinforcement Added criteria to EHR	Decreased CAUTI incidence rate from 3 to 1 (0.77% to 0.35% occurrence) 27.5% fewer patients with IUCs 20% decrease in catheter days 1 y after study compliance with: Indication: 100% Positioning: 100% Tamper-evident seal: 87.5% Securement device: 0% Team leader with support from MDs and nursing leadership contribute to success
Parry et al,[11] 2013	Aim to reduce IUC use and CAUTIs on all units Daily part of RN charting in EHR using protocol CPOE order for Foley mapped to nursing care Device-specific charting tool to address IUC presence and indications, and address removal plan Biweekly catheter use rates and CAUTI rates Used silver hydrogel urinary catheters, securement device optional, sealed drainage bag Bladder scanners used to assess urinary retention	Use of IUCs was reduced by 50.2% CAUTI rates reduced by 3.3% per month per catheter day and 5.29% per patient day Protocol changed culture; enhanced teamwork and ownership among the disciplines involved Nurse managers presented and discussed their unit rates, which increased institutional awareness and unit competition Estimated $100,000 savings and 6 lives Foley-free days in ICU

(continued on next page)

Table 1 (continued)		
Reference	Methodology	Overall Findings
Olson-Sitki et al,[8] 2015	Studied perceptions of a nurse-driven protocol to remove UCs without MD order 4 mo after implementation of protocol Anonymous Survey Monkey included a waiver as consent Scale was better, worse or no impact	20% decrease in catheter use after implementation of protocol Only half (53%) of the RNs used the protocol Job ease: 71% higher for users Empowerment: 80% of all Job satisfaction: no difference Patient feedback: 80% for users vs 20% for nonusers Physician feedback: no difference Younger RNs likely to use because of EBP in nursing school and openness to change in practice Job ease and efficiency of nursing work flow is integral to success

Abbreviations: CHG, chlorhexidine gluconate; CPOE, computerized provider order entry; CUCIS, Continued Urinary Catheter Indication Sheet; EHR, electronic health record; FIRM, Foley insertion removal maintenance; HOUDINI, hematuria, obstruction, urologic surgery, decubitus ulcer, I&O, no code, immobility; ICU, intensive care unit; TRIP, translating research into practice; UC, urinary catheter.

improved patient outcomes that included decreased IUC use, fewer catheter days, or a reduction in CAUTI rates. The quality improvement projects showed an increased nursing awareness of IUCs and introduced EBP based on current HICPAC guidelines to prevent CAUTIs. The research consistently showed how staff nurse engagement and nursing leadership were essential to successful outcomes.

NURSE EMPOWERMENT

Nurse empowerment is a perception that nurses have toward their practice environment,[8] and, not surprisingly, there is a correlation between job satisfaction and the quality of care.[8] For this project, this concept was operationalized using Kanter's theory of organizational empowerment. Kanter's theory guides nurse leaders to "create the conditions for nurses' work by shaping the quality of support, information, and resources available in work areas. When nurses perceive their leaders as authentic, open, and truthful and involve them in decision making, nurses respond positively to their work, reporting higher work engagement and greater trust in management."[16] The Theory comprises 6 concepts: formal power, informal power, access to information, access to support, access to resources, and opportunities for advancement[17,18] (**Fig. 1**). In order to implement the practice change, the theory provided structure, and the nurses collaborated on the plans, became active participants in the execution of the algorithm, and were responsible for the measured outcomes.

VISUAL MANAGEMENT

In the lean continuous process improvement model, the concept of visual management improves effective communication and promotes a reaction to change.[19] Boards that are centrally located, contain information that is relevant to the change process, show improvement is occurring, are easy to update, and incorporate staff ownership are effective visual management tools.[20] Two boards were used as visual

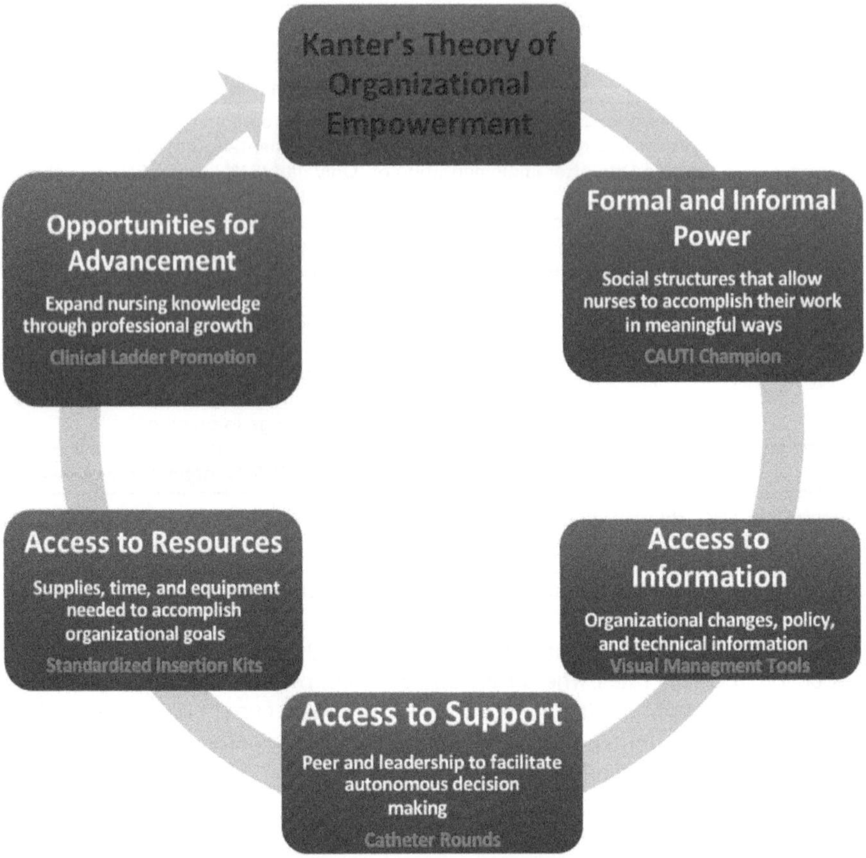

Fig. 1. Kanter's Theory of Organizational Empower was the guiding framework for this project. The 6 concepts are in large print, followed by their definition, and the green text are the concepts that were operationalized to effectively change nursing practice. (*Data from* Kanter RM. Men and women of the corporation. 2nd edition. New York: Basic Books; 1993.)

management tools for this project. The patient census board, located at the nurses' station, lists every patient's name and was used to identify patients with IUCs through the creation of Foley urinary catheter magnets (**Fig. 2**). The project status bulletin board, located within the nurses' station, provided information about the project, laminated copies of the algorithm, weekly graphs of IUC indications, weekly graphs by primary medical service, and examples of CAUTI reduction best practices (see "How the Protocol Works" at: https://infectionprevention.mednet.ucla.edu/files/view/education/CAUTI.pdf).

PROJECT DESIGN

The project design used the Model for Improvement (MFI). The MFI was selected because it has been used in many countries to successfully improve health care processes and outcomes.[21] The model comprises 2 equally important parts: the "thinking part," which comprises 3 fundamental questions that guide the change (**Table 2**), and the "doing part," which is a series of small change cycles using Plan, Do, Study, Act (PDSA) cycles.[22]

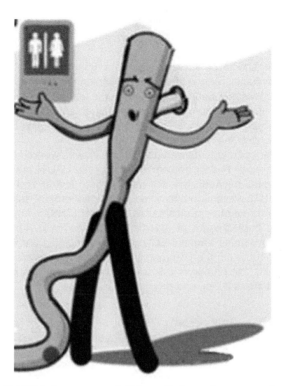

Fig. 2. An example of visual management. Foley catheter cartoon magnets were placed next to patient names on the patient census board and incorporated in data reports located on the project status bulletin board. (*Courtesy of* GiggleMed.com.)

The practice change was implemented during a 6-week period. Change was measured through daily audits, placement of magnets on the unit census board, and improved clinical assessment of appropriate use of IUCs. Nurses were instructed to remove the magnet when they removed the urinary catheter. The nurse leader performed daily catheter audits Monday through Friday to monitor appropriate

Table 2
The Model for Improvement was used to design the project structure, guide each new Plan, Do, Study, Act cycle, and keep the project team focused on the project goals

Question[21]	Definition[21]	Operationalized
(1) What are we trying to accomplish?	What will be changed, how will it be measured, and what results will occur because of this change?	Nursing management of IUCs Daily audits A 50% decrease in CAUTI incident rates from 4.80 to 2.40 per 1000 catheter days
(2) How will we know that a change is an improvement?	Data collection and quantitative measurements	An 80% algorithm use rate
(3) What change can we make that will result in improvement?	Input from stakeholders to determine plan of action using PDSA cycles	Education using visual management tools, daily catheter rounds, and trial of IUC removal algorithm

indications of IUCs. Audit data were collected using pen and paper, entered into an Excel spreadsheet, analyzed, and displayed on a project status bulletin board for staff to review.

Each PDSA cycle should be implemented on a small scale to allow for an easier start, provide rapid results, reduce the impact of unplanned effects, and allow a return to the previous processes if necessary.[22] The nurse leader met each week with the unit-based CAUTI champion nurse, reviewed the audit sheets, discussed any areas in need of improvement, and provided a report in the unit-based weekly update newsletter. **Table 3** describes the results of the PDSA cycles.

The primary project participants were the 38 nurses who worked between 7 AM and 7:30 PM Monday through Friday. Implementation of the CAUTI prevention algorithm was a shared process between the unit-based nurse leader and 1 bedside nurse who is the unit CAUTI prevention champion. Additional project assistance was provided by the CAUTI prevention clinical nurse specialist (CNS).

The project was implemented at a tertiary care academic medical center. The 45-bed adult cardiovascular thoracic SDU provides medical care for patients under the cardiology, vascular, lung, and transplant services. Nurses are assigned to 3 or 4 patients each shift. The primary medical providers are physicians, resident physicians, nurse practitioners (NPs), and physician assistants.

DATA TOOLS

Fig. 3 shows the audit tool used to measure catheter days, appropriate use of the algorithm, and IUC indication, and to record observation notes. Data collection started with a review of the daily census to determine which patients had IUCs. Nurses were identified by their initials. Catheter days was the total number of days that patients had an IUC divided by the number of days they were in the hospital.[6,13] The use of the CAUTI prevention algorithm data consisted of a manual review of the EHR and the nurse being asked to explain the clinical indication for the IUC during daily catheter rounds. If the patient met an algorithm criterion, a Y for yes or an N for no was marked in the appropriate audit tool column. The project team reviewed the EHR to ensure the IUC was removed and marked a Y for yes or N for no. The CAUTI incidence rate was calculated by taking the number of CAUTI infections, dividing it by the number of catheter days, and then multiplying by 1000.[13,15]

The project used charts and graphs to track the project's progress toward meeting the objective of 80% algorithm use. Displayed on the project status bulletin board, a run chart (**Fig. 4**) tracked the number of patients and use of the urinary catheter removal algorithm. Arrows were used to identify new PDSA cycles. Catheter use data by clinical indication (**Fig. 5**) and medical service (**Fig. 6**) were collected in the daily catheter rounds and displayed as observation pie graphs. The CAUTI incident rate results were charted on a line graph and reported to staff (**Fig. 7**). Before the project implementation, the CAUTI incidence rate was 4.80 per 1000 catheter days. The goal was to reduce the CAUTI rate by 50% following the implementation of the project. Zero CAUTIs occurred in May and June, but, because of the high number of infections earlier in the fiscal year, the incident rate showed a steady decrease from 4.80 in January 2017 to 3.05 in May 2017 (see **Fig. 7**).

DATA RESULTS

The nurse-driven algorithm to remove urinary catheters was used to educate the nurses about the change in clinical practice. Compliance with the algorithm was measured on accurate assessment and attainment of appropriate removal order.

Table 3
Plan, Do, Study, Act cycles used to implement the nurse-driven catheter-associated urinary tract infection prevention protocol

Stage	Definition	First Cycle	Second Cycle	Third Cycle
Plan	Objectives and predictions Who, what, when, where, and what data?[23]	Low algorithm use One-to-one education Increased IUC awareness Weekly report of data	Include voiding education and encourage earlier bladder scanning. Posted EBP examples on project status board	Tracked number of patients who were recatheterized and sent home with urology follow-up by service line
Do	Implementation of the test of change. All observations are documented for improvement and data are recorded and analyzed[23]	Conducted daily audits of nurses and reviewed EHR to identify barriers to IUC removal	Encouraged RNs to bladder scan patient 4 h after IUC removal instead of waiting 6 h to promote earlier voiding	Educated nurse about early intervention for surgical patients possibly experiencing postoperative urinary retention
Study	Data analyzed and compared with predictions. Reflections used to determine Act part of the cycle[23]	Compared baseline and study data. Found RNs bladder scanning patients at end of voiding trials	Found that patients were being recatheterized multiple times and discharged with an IUC	Vascular surgical patients with no history of retention were requiring urology follow-up
Act	Repeat the same cycle, modify the current cycle, or develop different cycles[22,23]	Continue with catheter rounds but include voiding education and encourage earlier bladder scanning	Continue with catheter rounds but encourage nurses to insert temporary catheters, bladder scan more frequently, and ask for medication orders to address urinary retention	Continue reinforcing early IUC removal and work with organization to implement removal algorithm for all nurses

Nurse-Driven Catheter Removal Algorithm Audit Tool							
Audit Date	Medical Record Number	Catheter Days	Algorithm Applicable (Y/N)	Algorithm Used (Y/N)	IUC Indication	RN Initials	Observation Notes

Fig. 3. Audit tool used to monitor daily use of the nurse-driven catheter removal algorithm. (*Courtesy of* Amy Larsen, CNS, San Francisco, CA.)

There were 54 patients with IUCs during the 6 weeks of the project. Of those patients, 31 patients met the algorithm criteria and their IUCs were removed before the end of the day shift at 7:30 PM. Even though the overall 57% compliance rate does not meet the project goal of 80%, it indicates a positive change in practice toward timely catheter removal.

One of the measurable objectives of this project was to reduce the CAUTI incidence rate by 50% from 4.80 to 2.40 per 1000 catheter days. At the time of the project implementation, there were 5 CAUTIs for the 2016 fiscal year (July 1, 2016, to June 30, 2017), therefore, the numerator in the CAUTI incident rate formula was 5. The hospital-wide infection control department calculated 119 catheter days in April 2017 and 136 catheter days in May 2017. The CAUTI rate was 3.32 per 1000 catheter days in April 2017 and 3.05 per 1000 catheter days in May 2017. The May 2017 CAUTI incident rate is a 37% reduction, which does not meet the project goal of 50% but is a positive indication of the change in CAUTI prevention nursing practice.

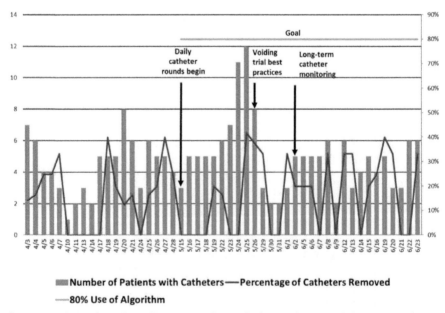

Fig. 4. Run chart of number of patients with IUCs before and during the project implementation. The arrows indicate the project implementation start date and initiation of new PDSA cycles.

RESULTS OF DAILY ROUNDS

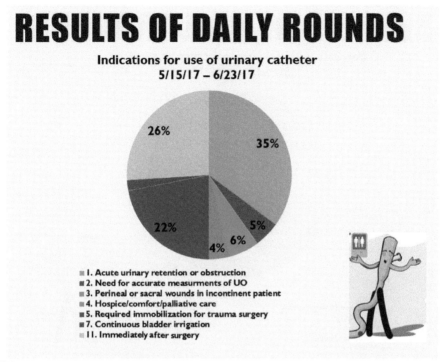

Indications for use of urinary catheter
5/15/17 – 6/23/17

- 1. Acute urinary retention or obstruction
- 2. Need for accurate measurments of UO
- 3. Perineal or sacral wounds in incontinent patient
- 4. Hospice/comfort/palliative care
- 5. Required immobilization for trauma surgery
- 7. Continuous bladder irrigation
- 11. Immediately after surgery

Fig. 5. Results of urinary catheter indications based on responses collected during daily catheter rounds. Weekly graphs were posted on the project status bulletin boards. UO, urinary output.

The daily catheter audits revealed trends in catheter days that required action plans via the PDSA cycles (see **Table 3**). Because catheter days are calculated by the number of days patients have an IUC, those patients with long-term IUCs significantly affect catheter day numbers if they have long hospitalizations. By the third week of the project, the number of patients with IUCs declined significantly and by the end of the week only 1 patient had a need for a long-term IUC. During the fourth week of the project, the number of catheter days continued to decrease and there were only 2 patients with long-term IUCs. In the fifth week of the project, on average, 3 patients per day had an IUC and only 1 patient required a long-term IUC.

Observable data, such as IUC indication (see **Fig. 5**) and service line (see **Fig. 6**), were displayed on the project status bulletin boards for the nursing staff to review. Service line data (see **Fig. 6**) brought awareness to nurses about which types of patients are likely to have an IUC and be at risk for a CAUTI. The indication data (see **Fig. 5**) highlighted nursing-assessed indications for an IUC, prompted the nurses to question unusual clinical indications, and referenced the removal algorithm for appropriate provider orders. These observations were important because they allowed the staff and providers to be more visually aware of the CAUTI prevention practices for at-risk patients.

The institution's nursing policy described 12 indications for use of urinary catheters (**Box 1**), which are similar to the HICPAC guidelines. Although nurses were required to document a daily assessment need of all IUCs, they did not have to indicate the indication. During daily catheter rounds, the nurse was asked to assess an indication

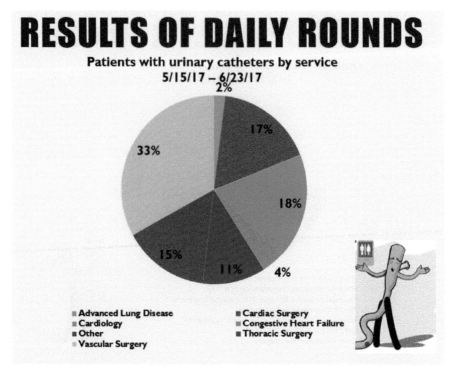

RESULTS OF DAILY ROUNDS
Patients with urinary catheters by service
5/15/17 – 6/23/17

2%
17%
33%
18%
15%
11%
4%

- Advanced Lung Disease
- Cardiology
- Other
- Vascular Surgery
- Cardiac Surgery
- Congestive Heart Failure
- Thoracic Surgery

Fig. 6. Graphic depiction of data by primary medical service representing the percentage of patients with urinary catheters. Weekly graphs were posted on the project status bulletin board. The "Other" category includes patients from the general surgery, malignant hematology, hospital medicine and orthopedics services who were admitted to the cardiovascular thoracic SDU for temporary placement.

using the list in **Box 1**. These data were collated and displayed on the project status bulletin board (see **Fig. 5**). During the project implementation, only 7 of the 12 indications were assessed on the cardiovascular thoracic SDU (see **Fig. 5**). Although immediately after surgery was highly used (26% of patients), many of these patients were managed by surgical NPs who wrote IUC discontinuation orders early in the day following their morning patient rounds, which was the essence of the EBP algorithm.

As part of this project, the CNS asked the project team to identify a high-IUC use service line. Once identified, the unit could collaborate with providers to include the algorithm in their standard patient orders. Data compiled weekly indicated that the vascular surgical team was the best service to implement this change (see **Fig. 6**). The heart failure service had a low number of patients, which relates to the low use of IUCs for strict measurement of urinary output. This finding indicates the use of other methods to calculate urine output, such as metered urinals and urine catch devices placed in patient bathrooms.

RELATIONSHIP OF RESULTS TO THE FRAMEWORK, AIMS, AND OBJECTIVES

The guiding framework for this project was Kanter's theory of organizational empowerment (see **Fig. 1**). As the results show, this framework was effective in empowering the staff nurses to change their CAUTI prevention practices. They actively participated

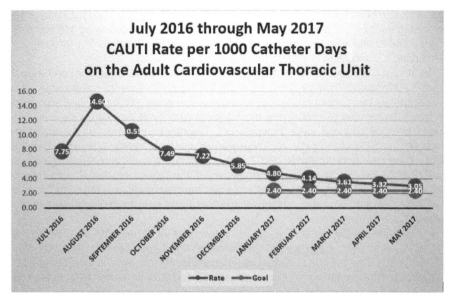

Fig. 7. CAUTI infection for the fiscal year 2017. There was 1 infection in July, 4 infections in August, and 1 infection in November. Data are per 1000 catheter days. The goal reflects the project aim to reduce the CAUTI rate by 50% from 4.80 to 2.40.

in the project through collaboration with providers to remove IUCs. During catheter rounds, nurses shared CAUTI prevention practices from previous nursing jobs. In addition, they took an active role in visual awareness of IUCs through use of the Foley magnets on the patient census board. After the first 2 weeks of the project, the nurses became more familiar with the 12 urinary catheter indications, which decreased the

---

Box 1
Organizational list of approved indications for use of urinary catheter

1. Acute urinary retention or obstruction

2. Need for accurate measurements of urinary output in critically ill patients

3. Perineal or sacral wounds in incontinent patients

4. Hospice/comfort/palliative care

5. Required immobilization for trauma surgery

6. Patients undergoing urologic surgery

7. Patients with continuous bladder irrigation

8. Foley needed for medication administration

9. Chronic indwelling catheter present on admission

10. Patient undergoing prolonged (>2 hours) procedure

11. Immediately after surgery (plan to discontinue within time frame as ordered)

12. Other (specify)

If the patient does not have any of the indications the RN is to notify the provider to discuss plan for removal.

---

time it took to complete daily catheter rounds. They proactively placed the Foley magnets on the patient census board and promptly removed them following IUC removal. The nurses identified this project as a unit-based quality improvement project and referenced it during new graduate nurse interviews.

The aim of the project was to implement a CAUTI prevention algorithm and reduce the CAUTI incidence rate by 50%. Although the algorithm was not implemented into nursing policy because of challenges to the provider order set, it provided an opportunity for the nurses to experience the full responsibility of IUC care when the proposed practice changes were implemented. The results showed that the algorithm was used for 57% of the patients. There was an unexpected high number of patients with urinary retention problems, and 7 of the 54 patients were discharged home with an IUC and urology consultation appointment. Even though the CAUTI rate did not decrease by 50% from 4.80 to 2.40 per 1000 catheter days, the May 2017 rate of 3.04 reflected a 36% change, which is significant and reflects the increased awareness of IUCs among the staff.

The objectives were met and resulted in increased CAUTI prevention education, the trial of the algorithm, daily catheter audits, reporting of audit results, use of the MFI, and comparison of the CAUTI rates before and after the project. Although data analysis assisted in identifying nursing practices around IUC care, the MFI allowed for changes to the project plan through the initiation of each new PDSA cycle. Despite modifications to the objectives, the results showed that there was significant effort in achieving the desired outcomes.

IMPACT OF RESULTS ON PRACTICE

The success of this project brought a new enthusiasm for nursing-sensitive outcomes to the cardiovascular thoracic SDU nursing staff. The project raised awareness of clinical practice standards and critically assessing patients with IUCs. This change in practice and the success of reducing CAUTIs is something the nurses were proud of when describing unit-based initiatives.

The use of visual management tools affected the attainment of the objectives. The Foley catheter magnets aided in quickly determining the number of patients with IUCs; provided a reminder to staff entering the patients' rooms to be mindful of the IUCs; and, anecdotally, the nurses who removed the IUCs were rewarded with taking the magnet off the patient census board. The project status bulletin board, an effective communication tool, kept the staff up to date on the project progress and all materials were laminated so they would remain intact after the project implementation. Information was easy to create using PowerPoint, simple to update, and will be used as the template for future quality improvement projects on the unit.

The daily catheter rounds were empowering to the CAUTI prevention champion and educational to the nurse leader. By the end of the second week of the project, the staff proactively anticipated audits of all their patients with IUCs. They were educational for the nurse leader in that they provided an opportunity to learn about challenges the nurses had with providers, and about best practices from other health care organizations, and to gain a better appreciation for IUCs in the patient population.

STRENGTHS AND LIMITATIONS OF THE PROJECT

The primary strength of this project was the implementation of EBP CAUTI prevention practices. The use of Foley magnets on the patient census boards as visual management reminders and the adoption of the cartoon urinary catheter improved effective communication and encouraged awareness of catheter clinical assessment.[6,7,10,11]

The proposed catheter removal algorithm was shown to decrease catheter days and will likely be implemented into practice.[1] The daily catheter audits were evidence that consistent nursing leadership presence empowers staff nurses to provide the best care.[15]

This project was limited by organizational policies that did not allow for the implementation of the urinary catheter removal algorithm. The nurses were required to use the tool to assess for urinary catheter appropriateness but still needed to collaborate with the providers to remove the IUC. Although the project team consistently completed the daily catheter rounds, they were not always performed at the same time of day. Ideally, the daily catheter rounds should have occurred at 7:30 AM following the nurse handoff so that collaboration with providers for IUC removal could happen early in the day. More often, the daily catheter rounds occurred later in the day when the project team and staff nurses were available to discuss this plan of care. The final limitation was the number of patients with IUCs on the cardiovascular thoracic SDU. On average, there were only 3 to 4 patients with IUCs, which made it challenging to achieve the project aim of a 50% CAUTI incident rate reduction.

FUTURE IMPLICATIONS FOR PRACTICE

Although the CAUTI incidence rate was trending downward, the implementation of a CAUTI prevention algorithm allowed the nurse leader to identify other practice areas in need of improvement. During this project, she realized that the organization lacks a voiding trial algorithm. Although there are standard orders for nurses to contact the provider if the patient does not void within 6 hours of urinary catheter removal, there are no interventions the nurse can reference to encourage voiding. Another area of practice that needs to be addressed is urinary retention in postoperative vascular patients. The project team will work with the vascular service NPs to find ways to avoid urinary retention before the removal of the IUC. In addition, this project will serve as an example of the ease of implementing EBP at the bedside in hopes that it will inspire staff nurses to improve nursing outcomes on the unit level and throughout the organization.

REFERENCES

1. Timmons B, Vess J, Conner B. Nurse-driven protocol to reduce indwelling catheter dwell time: a health care improvement initiative. J Nurs Care Qual 2017; 32(2):104–7.
2. Gould C. Catheter-associated urinary tract infection (CAUTI) toolkit. Available at: http://www.cdc.gov/HAI/pdfs/toolkits/CAUTItoolkit_3_10.pdf. Accessed September 25, 2016.
3. Peasch SK, McKay NL, Harman JS, et al. Medicare non-payment of hospital-acquired infections: infection rates three years post implementation. Medicare Medicaid Res Rev 2013;3(3):1–13. Available at: https://www.cms.gov/mmrr/Downloads/MMRR2013_003_03_a08.pdf. Accessed November 12, 2016.
4. Healthcare Infection Control Practices Advisory Committee. Guideline for prevention of catheter-associated urinary tract infections 2009. Available at: http://www.cdc.gov/HAI/ca_uti/uti.html. Accessed September 25, 2016.
5. Zimlichman E, Henderson D, Tamir O, et al. Health care–associated infections a meta-analysis of costs and financial impact on the US health care system. JAMA Intern Med 2013;173(22):2039–46.
6. Mori C. A-voiding catastrophe: implementing a nurse-driven protocol. Medsurg Nurs 2014;23(1):15–28.

7. Gokula M, Smolen D, Gaspar PM, et al. Designing a protocol to reduce catheter-associated urinary tract infections among hospitalized patients. Am J Infect Control 2012;40(2012):1002–4.

8. Olson-Sitki K, Kirkbride G, Forbes G. Evaluation of a nurse-driven protocol to remove urinary catheters: nurses' perceptions. Urol Nurs 2015;35(2):94–9.

9. Melnyk BM, Fineout-Overholt E. Evidence-based practice in nursing & healthcare: a guide to best practice. Philadelphia: Lippincott Williams & Wilkins; 2015. p. 604.

10. Andreessen L, Wilde MH, Herendeen P. Preventing catheter-associated urinary tract infections in acute care. J Nurs Care Qual 2012;27(3):209–17.

11. Parry MF, Grant B, Sestovic M. Successful reduction in catheter-associated urinary tract infections: Focus on nurse-directed catheter removal. Am J Infect Control 2013;41(2013):1178–81.

12. Johnson P, Gilman A, Lintner A, et al. Nurse-driven catheter associated urinary tract infection reduction process and protocol: development through an academic-practice partnership. Crit Care Nurs Q 2016;39(4):352–62.

13. Marra AR, Camargo TZ, Goncalves P, et al. Preventing catheter-associated urinary tract infection in the zero-tolerance era. Am J Infect Control 2011;39(10): 817–22.

14. Oman KS, Makic MBF, Fink R, et al. Nurse-directed interventions to reduce catheter-associated urinary tract infections. Am J Infect Control 2012;40(2012): 548–53.

15. Underwood L. The effect of implementing a comprehensive unit-based safety program on urinary catheter use. Urol Nurs 2015;35(6):271–9.

16. Wong CA, Laschinger HKS. Authentic leadership, performance, and job satisfaction: The mediating role of empowerment. J Adv Nurs 2012;69(4):947–59.

17. Skytt B, Hagerman H, Stromberg A, et al. First-line managers' descriptions and reflections regarding their staff's access to empowering structures. J Nurs Manag 2015;23(8):1003–10.

18. Laschinger HKS, Fida R. Linking nurses' perceptions of patient care quality to job satisfaction: The role of authentic leadership and empowering professional practice environments. J Nurs Adm 2015;45(5):276–83.

19. Six sigma material. Visual management. Available at: http://www.six-sigma-material.com/Visual-Management.html. Accessed February 15, 2017.

20. Total Excellence Manufacturing (TXM). Five tips to designing and effective team visual management board. Available at: http://txm.com.au/blog/five-tips-designing-effective-team-visual-management-board. Accessed February 15, 2017.

21. Institute for Healthcare Improvement. Model for Improvement. Available at: http://www.ihi.org/resources/PublishingImages/ModelforImprovement.jpg. Accessed February 17, 2017.

22. Care Inspectorate. Tool 20a: the Model for Improvement. Available at: http://www.careinspectorate.com/images/documents/2737/Tool_20a.pdf. Accessed February 13, 2017.

23. Institute for Healthcare Improvement. The PDSA cycle for learning and improving. Available at: http://www.ihi.org/resources/PublishingImages/PDSA.jpg. Accessed February 17, 2017.

Evaluation of Telemetry Utilization on Medical-Surgical Units

JoAnne Phillips, DNP, RN, CNS, CPPS[a],*,
Rosemary C. Polomano, PhD, RN[b],
Treasa 'Susie' Leming-Lee, DNP, MSN, RN[c],
Terri Davis Crutcher, DNP, MSN, RN[d]

KEYWORDS

- Alarm fatigue • Telemetry utilization • Clinical alarms • Alarm safety

KEY POINTS

- Alarm fatigue is the leading cause of alarm-related patient harm. Nurses that experience alarm fatigue may ignore, disable, or delay response to alarms.
- The American Heart Association (AHA) guidelines for telemetry monitoring recommend which patients should be monitored and for what period of time.
- Research on telemetry monitoring outside the intensive care unit demonstrate there is a 35% overuse of telemetry monitoring, which may result in excessive alarms, contributing to alarm fatigue.
- Understanding nurse's perceptions of alarms and alarm fatigue related to telemetry may help to develop an improvement plan. Nurse's attitudes and practices related to alarm safety were evaluated.

INTRODUCTION

The use of complex monitoring technology in clinical environments has increased significantly over the past three decades. In 1983, critical care units averaged six different types of monitoring devices with clinical alarms, and by 2011 that number rose to 40.[1,2] Most clinical alarms alert clinicians to either a change in the patient's physiologic status or a problem with the equipment.[3–6] Patients on physiologic monitors experience an average of 350 to 700 alarms per patient per day.[4–7] Noise generated by alarms is disruptive and anxiety producing for health care providers resulting

Disclosure Statement: Neither author has anything to disclose.
[a] Virtua Health System, 303 Lippincott Drive, Suite 200, Marlton, NJ 08053, USA; [b] University of Pennsylvania School of Nursing, University of Pennsylvania Perelman School of Medicine, 418 Curie Boulevard, Philadelphia, PA 19104, USA; [c] Vanderbilt University School of Nursing, 461 21st Avenue South, 216 Godchaux Hall, Nashville, TN 37240, USA; [d] Vanderbilt University School of Nursing, 222 Godchaux Hall, 461 21st Avenue South, Nashville, TN 37240, USA
* Corresponding author.
E-mail address: jphillips3@virtua.org

Nurs Clin N Am 54 (2019) 97–114
https://doi.org/10.1016/j.cnur.2018.10.001
0029-6465/19/© 2018 Elsevier Inc. All rights reserved.

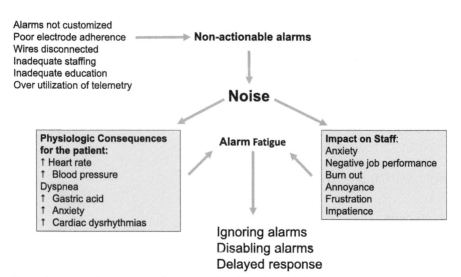

Alarms not customized
Poor electrode adherence ⟶ **Non-actionable alarms**
Wires disconnected
Inadequate staffing
Inadequate education
Over utilization of telemetry

Noise

Physiologic Consequences for the patient:	**Alarm Fatigue**	**Impact on Staff:**
↑ Heart rate		Anxiety
↑ Blood pressure		Negative job performance
Dyspnea		Burn out
↑ Gastric acid		Annoyance
↑ Anxiety		Frustration
↑ Cardiac dysrhythmias		Impatience

Ignoring alarms
Disabling alarms
Delayed response

Fig. 1. Concept of the impact of noise on the physiology of the patient, and the impact on staff. (*Data from* Hsu SM, Ko WJ, Liao WC, et al. Associations of exposure to noise with physiological and psychological outcomes among post-cardiac surgery patients in ICUs. Clinics (Sao Paulo) 2010;65(10):985–9; and Hsu T, Ryherd E, Waye KP, et al. Noise pollution in hospitals: impact on patients. J Clin Outcomes Manag 2012;19(7):301–9.)

in a syndrome referred to as alarm fatigue (**Fig. 1**). Alarm fatigue is the "limited capacity to identify and prioritize alarm signals, which has led to delayed or failed alarm responses and deliberate alarm deactivations."[8] Alarm fatigue poses a significant risk to patient safety, and is the most common contributing factor in alarm-related sentinel events.[9] Nurses experiencing alarm fatigue may disable, silence, or ignore clinical alarms placing patients at risk for experiencing a change in their health status requiring immediate interventions.[5,10]

Nonactionable and nuisance alarms are key contributors to alarm fatigue. Nonactionable alarms result from a violation of an alarm parameter that does not require patient therapeutic intervention. Nuisance alarms refer to the occurrence of a high number of nonactionable alarms.[11] Nonactionable alarms related to telemetry monitoring result from inadequate individualized customization of alarm parameter ranges, disconnection of lead wires, inadequate staff education and nurse staffing resources, improper management of electrodes, or the use of telemetry monitoring outside of evidence-based practice guidelines.[5–7,10,12,13] Both clinical and technical deficiencies lead to alarm fatigue, which is addressed by consistent standards of practice, education and competency assessments, and technical standardization (**Fig. 2**). The "Practice Standards for Electrocardiographic Monitoring in Hospital Settings" by Drew and colleagues[14] are evidence-based practice guidelines supported by the American Heart Association (AHA) to guide clinicians in selecting appropriate patients for continuous electrocardiographic or cardiac monitoring and the duration of such monitoring. The AHA recommends using patient selection criteria in three categories (class I, II, and III) to determine indications and benefits for the appropriate use of cardiac monitoring (**Table 1**). The overuse of telemetry as a cause of nonactionable alarms despite the availability of these evidence-based national practice standards for defining patient selection prompted a project to examine telemetry use and practice patterns for provider orders and discontinuation of telemetry monitoring in a medical-surgical setting.

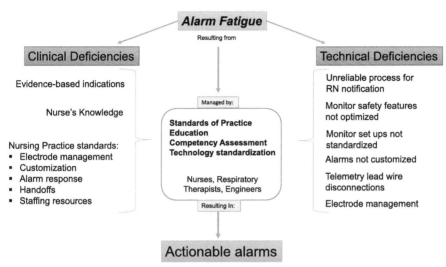

Fig. 2. Concept of alarm fatigue. (*Data from* Refs.[2,5–7,10,12])

BACKGROUND

Since 2007, the ECRI Institute, an independent nonprofit organization researching approaches to improving patient care, has published a list of the top health care technology hazards with alarm hazards remaining at or near the top of the list.[15–21] Alarm-related harm data are reported through several data bases, including, but not limited to, the Manufacturer and User Facility Device experience (MAUDE) database of the Food and Drug Administration (FDA) and The Joint Commission (TJC) sentinel event program. MAUDE is a database of adverse event reports submitted to the FDA by manufacturers, importers, and device users. From 2005 to 2010, there were 566 reports of alarm-related deaths entered into the MAUDE database.[9,22,23] Follow-up investigations revealed that clinicians using monitoring equipment were unfamiliar with how the monitoring equipment worked or failed to checked the monitor's alarm status.[22] TJC defines a sentinel event as "an unexpected occurrence involving death or serious physical or psychological injury, or the risk thereof."[24] From 2009 to 2012, a total of 98 alarm-related sentinel events were reported to TJC, which resulted in 80 patient deaths, 13 patients with permanent loss of function, and five patients requiring unexpected additional care or extended hospitalization.[9] Sentinel event reporting to TJC is voluntary, thus it is likely that alarm-related sentinel events are underreported.[2,6,9,23]

Alarm fatigue is the most common factor contributing to alarm-related patient harm. Inappropriate use or overuse of telemetry monitoring is a key factor in alarm fatigue. The gold standard for use of telemetry monitoring is the "Practice Standards for Electrocardiographic Monitoring in Hospital Settings" by Drew and colleagues[14] and endorsed by the AHA. However, researchers report that telemetry practices are often not aligned with the AHA guidelines.[12,25–29] More than three-quarters (85%–99%) of clinical alarms are nonactionable and considered nuisance alarms; a significant problem leading to alarm fatigue.[5,7,10,12,13] Nurses can spend 16% to 35% of patient care time responding to alarms.[4,13,30] The noise from nuisance alarms can overwhelm health care providers making it difficult to discriminate between alarm sounds and prioritize alarms that require an immediate response.

Table 1 Telemetry practice guidelines	
Classification	**Descriptors**

Class I Electrocardiogram monitoring is indicated in most, if not all, patients in this group Patients at significant risk of a life-threatening arrhythmia	• Postcardiac resuscitation
	• Early phase of acute coronary syndromes
	• Unstable coronary syndromes and newly diagnosed coronary lesions
	• Adults and children after cardiac surgery
	• Nonurgent percutaneous coronary intervention with complications
	• Patients in critical care
	• Patients with
	  ○ An implantation of an automatic defibrillator or a permanent pacemaker and are considered pacer dependent; have a temporary pacemaker or transcutaneous pacing pads
	  ○ Atrioventricular block; arrhythmias complicated Wolff-Parkinson-White syndrome
	  ○ With long-QT syndrome and associated ventricular arrhythmias
	  ○ Intra-aortic balloon pump
	  ○ Acute heart failure/pulmonary edema
	  ○ Undergoing moderate sedation
	  ○ Hemodynamic unstable arrhythmias
	  ○ Arrhythmias in pediatric patients

Class II Cardiac monitoring may be of benefit in some patients but is not considered essential for all patients	• Postacute myocardial infarction • Chest pain syndromes • Uncomplicated, nonurgent percutaneous coronary interventions • Receiving antiarrhythmic drugs • Pacemaker insertion, not pacer dependent • Uncomplicated ablation • Uncomplicated coronary angiography • Subacute heart failure • Being evaluated for syncope • Do-not-resuscitate orders with arrhythmias that cause discomfort
Class III Cardiac monitoring is not indicated	• Low-risk postoperative patients • Obstetric patients, unless they have heart disease • Permanent rate controlled atrial fibrillation

American Heart Association guidelines for telemetry, 2004.[14]

Data from Drew BJ, Califf RM, Funk M, et al. AHA scientific statement: practice standards for electrocardiographic monitoring in hospital settings: an American Heart Association scientific statement from the Councils on Cardiovascular Nursing, Clinical Cardiology, and Cardiovascular Disease in the Young: endorsed by the International Society of Computerized Electrocardiology and the American Association of Critical-Care Nurses. J Cardiovasc Nurs 2005;20(2):76–106.

Impact of Alarm Fatigue

Alarm fatigue is an adaptive mechanism to manage the complex cognitive burden associated with alarms[31] but it is also a coping mechanism to manage the barrage of auditory or visual (eg, flashing) stimulation created by alarms. Nurses respond to alarms based on the perceived reliability of the alarm. Delayed responses to alarms not only evoke stress among patients, family members, and other caregivers, but more seriously lead to adverse clinical outcomes.[31] The noise associated with clinical alarms can have negative physiologic effects on patients, families, and staff (see **Fig. 1**).

Dressler and colleagues[26] implemented an evidence-based electronic order set for cardiac monitoring based on the AHA guidelines. This resulted in a 70% reduction in the mean daily number of patients monitored with telemetry, 357 to 109 patients, which was not associated with a notable change in cardiac arrest, rapid response, or hospital mortality metrics and translated into an estimated cost savings of $4.8 million in 1 year.[26] Benjamin and colleagues[25] and Dressler and colleagues[26] estimated the cost of telemetry to be $53 per day, but neither study captured manpower resources, such as telemetry or monitoring technicians versus nurse accountability models of care.

Review of Literature

For the scientific rationale to support a project examining patterns of telemetry use and adherence to evidence-based practice guidelines, a literature search was conducted using Pub Med, Cumulative Index of Nursing and Allied Health Literature, and Ovid. Key search terms were "alarm fatigue," "cardiac telemetry," "alarm safety," and "clinical alarms." The search was restricted to citations in English and human subjects only within the past 5 years. Article titles and abstracts were screened to ensure a focus on cardiac telemetry, telemetry use, and alarm fatigue. Supporting literature was compiled in the following areas.

Several studies document that the use of telemetry is inconsistent with the AHA guidelines.[12,26–29] Feder and Funk[12] analyzed telemetry utilization on 2766 patients in the PULSE trial, a multicenter, 5-year study that examined the relationship between nurse knowledge, education, and patient outcomes. In the PULSE trial, investigators found that 35% of days that patients were on telemetry were not indicated based on AHA guidelines. Benjamin and colleagues[25] corroborated this findings noting that of 1559 monitored days for 501 patients, 35% (548 days) were not supported by AHA guidelines.

Observational studies conducted by Gazarian and colleagues[31] and Gazarian[32] with the same data but different research questions explored nurses' behaviors and attitudes about responding to alarms. Authors concluded that acknowledging and responding to alarms requires cognitive processing involving recognizing how important the alarm is, how reliable it is, where it is coming from, and who else might be responding.[4,30–32] Overuse of telemetry is linked to alarm fatigue, excessive noise, increased length of hospital stay, emergency department boarding, ambulance diversion and operating costs, and decreased hospital throughput and decreased patient satisfaction.[6,7,10,25,33] Some authors contend that telemetry monitoring does not contribute to early detection of critical arrhythmias or clinical deterioration.[12,28,31,34] In contrast, Cleverley and colleagues[35] in a retrospective analysis of 668 patients after cardiac arrest from pulseless electrical activity or asystole documented better outcomes with initial resuscitation for patients on telemetry compared with no telemetry monitoring (66% vs 34%; $P = .02$) and improved survival to hospital discharge (30% vs 6%; $P = .01$).

Telemetry practices outlined in the AHA-endorsed "Practice Standards for Electrocardiographic Monitoring in Hospital Settings," whereas evidence-based by expert opinion, have limitations. Drew and colleagues[14] acknowledge that there is a lack of published clinical trials on hospital monitoring with decision-making for telemetry practices and recognize the need for consensus on cardiac monitoring. Although these guidelines were originally published in 2004, an updated report was published in 2017.[36] The 2017 guidelines still emphasize that 35% to 43% of patients monitored in non–intensive care unit settings have no clinical indication for monitoring. In addition, these new recommendations for telemetry primarily address cardiology patients, and include only a few recommendations for noncardiac patient populations. Previous work in process improvement for telemetry use shows tremendous practice variations in indications and duration for telemetry and uptake of the AHA guidelines to inform practices.[13,25,26,37–39] Henriques-Forsythe and colleagues[27] conducted a review of the literature that identified potential barriers to adherence to evidence-based guidelines. These include lack of awareness of the guidelines or nonadherence to the guidelines. Leighton and colleagues[40] hypothesized that electronic order sets for telemetry would improve compliance with the guidelines, which is consistent with Dressler and colleagues.[26] However after 48 hours, a high percentage of patients in Leighton's study that had electronic order sets remained on telemetry without an indication. Dressler and colleagues[26] hardwired a telemetry protocol based on the AHA guidelines into the electronic medical record (EMR), which also included a nurse-driven discontinuation protocol. This strategy demonstrated a sustained 43% decrease in telemetry initiation and a 70% overall reduction in telemetry use with no notable increase in mortality, cardiac arrest, or rapid response team activation.

Significant gaps exist in the foundational science for telemetry use and alarm management with most work in the area of telemetry use focused on process improvement. There is a lack of research examining customization of alarm settings, nurse's response to alarms, and perception and attitudes of nurses toward alarms. The literature is clear, however, that clinical environments are overwhelmed with monitoring device alarms, which have a negative effect on nurses, patients, and families. More studies are needed to guide nurses' clinical decision-making on how to customize alarms and mitigate risks associated with the overpowering number of nonactionable, false, or nuisance alarms. Despite accepted evidence-based practice guidelines for telemetry, barriers to uptake of these guidelines remain unclear, making it difficult to implement effective strategies to promote guideline concordant care. The specific aims of this project were to examine practice patterns related to ordering and discontinuing telemetry monitoring to determine if these were aligned with the AHA evidence-based practice guidelines; and to assess nurses' perceptions, issues, improvements, and priorities for alarm safety using the Healthcare Technology Foundation Survey on "Perceptions, Issues, Improvements, and Priorities of Healthcare Professionals" (http://thehtf.org/alarms_survey2011.asp).

METHODS
Design

This quality improvement project used the "define, measure, analyze, improve, and control" (DMAIC) methodology to identify and eliminate defects in processes or products.[41] The DMAIC model is recommended for processes that are complex or high risk.[42] This model-guided work to the Healthcare Technology Foundation (HTF) Survey on "Perceptions, Issues, Improvements, and Priorities of Healthcare Professionals" was administered to all registered nurses on the two study units to help to define staff attitudes and perceptions related to alarm safety. The Vanderbilt University Institutional Review Board and the University of Pennsylvania Institutional Review Board approved this project as exempt status.

Setting and Participants

This project was conducted on a 40-bed medical unit and a 32-bed surgical unit at the Hospital of the University of Pennsylvania (HUP), a 776-bed academic magnet-designated medical center located in Philadelphia, Pennsylvania. There are 16 medical-surgical units at HUP and all have the capability to monitor patients on telemetry, with the unit census ranging from 28 to 40 patients; the telemetry census can range from 0 to 24 patients. Although several sources discuss the difference in cost between a medical-surgical bed and a telemetry bed,[12,25,27,28] HUP does not charge for telemetry and there are no true telemetry units, so there is no revenue associated with telemetry. The cost avoidance is achieved through nursing and transport time.

The hospital has a fully integrated computerized provider order entry system and EMR. Telemetry monitoring for patients outside the intensive care units required a licensed provider (eg, physician or advanced practice provider [APPs; nurse practitioner or physician assistant]). Although the EMR includes a telemetry order set based on the AHA guidelines, other criteria specify additional indications not congruent with the AHA guidelines (**Table 2**). Each telemetry order defines a time indication, either 24 or 48 hours (or the duration of the treatment). A subsequent provider order must be written by the provider to discontinue telemetry monitoring, even if the time for the indication for monitoring is expired. To understand the financial impact of telemetry use at HUP, an understanding of the current state of the estimated cost of telemetry was essential. Before beginning this project, the two units selected for this project had an average of seven telemetry patients per day. Based on estimates from Feder and Funk[12] and Benjamin and colleagues,[25] of a 35% overuse of telemetry, the impact of aligning practice patterns with the evidence-based practice guidelines would result in a cost avoidance of an estimated $47,395 for each 40-bed medical-surgical unit. This project examined the relationship between the evidence-based guidelines, the patient's clinical status, and the use of telemetry.

Table 2 Electronic order set and the AHA guidelines		
Indication	**Hours**	**Class AHA**
AHA indications not included in the order set		
IABP	Duration	Class I
Moderate sedation	Duration	Class I
Antiarrhythmic drugs for rate control	Duration	Class II
Routine coronary angiography	24	Class II
DNR with dysrhythmias that cause discomfort	Duration	Class II
Indications in order set and not in AHA guidelines		
Atrial tachyarrhythmias, uncontrolled	48	
OSA, postoperative patients only	48	
Electrolyte imbalance (severe): potassium, magnesium, and calcium	24	
Postoperative state (not renewable for this indication)	24	

Abbreviations: DNR, do not resuscitate; IABP, intra-aortic balloon pump; OSA, obstructive sleep apnea.

Data from Drew BJ, Califf RM, Funk M, et al. AHA scientific statement: practice standards for electrocardiographic monitoring in hospital settings: an American Heart Association scientific statement from the Councils on Cardiovascular Nursing, Clinical Cardiology, and Cardiovascular Disease in the Young: endorsed by the International Society of Computerized Electrocardiology and the American Association of Critical-Care Nurses. J Cardiovasc Nurs 2005;20(2):76–106.

Process Improvement Methodology Using DMAIC

Define

The first step for this project required a charter to establish the scope of work, assemble a project team of nurse and physician leaders, and conduct a stakeholder analysis. The charter defined the problem, business case, problem statement, and goals, and identified project milestones with metrics to determine the success of the project. A work plan outlined the timeline for all activities and a process map detailed differences between the process for ordering or discontinuing telemetry on the two medical-surgical study units (**Fig. 3**).

Measure

During the 4-week study period, a total of 94 unique patients received provider orders for telemetry. To facilitate daily review of telemetry orders, a report summarizing all current telemetry orders was available from the EMR, and was printed out for each unit at 6:00 PM each day for 4 weeks. Based on the telemetry report, individual chart reviews were conducted for all patients on telemetry to facilitate the collection of required data. Data included the primary or principle diagnosis related to telemetry, indication for telemetry from the electronic order set, role of the provider who placed the order for telemetry, and AHA class for telemetry. All patient data were deidentified. The time difference between date and time of the initial order and the date and time of the discontinuation order were calculated.

The HTF survey "Perceptions, Issues, Improvements, and Priorities of Healthcare Professionals" measures attitudes and practices related to clinical alarms. Attitudes and practices may influence the unit culture regarding alarm safety. The survey was administered in 2006 and again in 2011 to a national sample of nurses, providers, respiratory therapists, and physical and occupational therapists across the country to assess attitudes and perceptions of clinical alarms. Responses between the initial

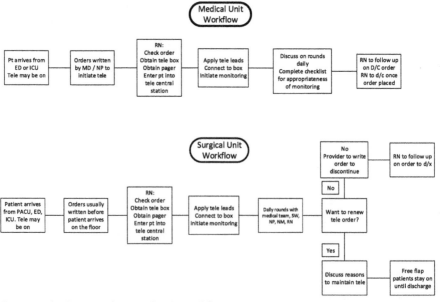

Fig. 3. Medical unit and surgical unit workflow.

2006 survey and subsequent 2011 survey did not show significant differences in the responses to the questions on attitudes and practices related to alarm safety.[43] For this project, the Healthcare Technology Foundation Survey administered to nurses on two units revealed important information about the attitudes and practices of clinical nurses related to alarms and alarm fatigue.

RESULTS
Analyze

The sample of 94 patients consisted of 58.5% (n = 55) men and 41.5% (n = 39) women with a mean age of 59.84 years (standard deviation, 14.3). There were 57 medical patients with 83% having orders written by physicians and 17% by APPs, and 37 surgical patients with 67% written by physicians and 33% by AAPs. Of these 94 patients with telemetry orders, 68% (64) were outside the AHA guidelines. The remaining orders were in class I (10%) and class II (22%). The most common indications for telemetry included electrolyte imbalance (21%), postoperative care (17%), and palpitations (17%) (**Table 3**), which together constituted 55% of the orders. None of these indications is recommended in the AHA guidelines.

The stated reasons for telemetry were congruent with the patient's clinical condition for 39 (43%) patients. A more in-depth chart review was conducted for patients with an indication for "severe electrolyte imbalance of potassium, calcium or magnesium" and for "QT prolonging medications." For the 20 (21%) patients with orders for severe electrolyte imbalance, the patient's electrolyte values in the 24 hours preceding the telemetry order were reviewed. If an electrolyte deficit was noted the provider orders were reviewed to assess for electrolyte replacement. Of the 20 patients with order for severe electrolyte imbalance, two patients had normal electrolytes; one patient did not have electrolytes ordered. Calcium disturbances were the most predominant abnormality, affecting 10 patients. Only one patient with hypokalemia met the organization's criteria for a critical laboratory value with a potassium value of 2.8 mmol/L.

Table 3 Telemetry orders		
Indication	**Number of Patients (%)**	**AHA Class**
Electrolytes	20 (21)	None
Postoperative	16 (17)	None
Palpitations	16 (17)	None
QT prolonging medications	7 (7)	II
Atrial tachyarrhythmias	6 (6)	None
CHF, active	4 (4)	II
Syncope	4 (4)	II
Intermediate-/high-risk chest pain	4 (4)	II
Stroke	3 (3)	None
Low-risk chest pain	3 (3)	II
Arrhythmias with unstable hemodynamics	3 (3)	I
Unrestricted	3 (3)	None
Unstable hemodynamics	2 (2)	I
Acute coronary syndrome	2 (2)	II
Critical care patient	1 (1)	I

Abbreviation: CHF, congestive heart failure.

Seven patients had orders for QT-prolonging medications. The QTc for seven patients was assessed by reviewing the interpretation on their 12-lead electrocardiograms. Only one patient had a QTc that was higher than the upper limit of normal of 470 milliseconds. Each patient's medications were reviewed and compared with the list of medications that not only prolong QTc intervals, but also place the patient at risk for torsades de pointes, a polymorphic ventricular tachycardia.[44] There were five medications prescribed for seven patients in this study that had high or intermediate risk to cause torsades de pointes. These medications included ondansetron and haloperidol (high risk), famotidine, metronidazole, and quetiapine (intermediate risk).[45] Ondansetron was prescribed for six of the seven patients. Ondansetron has a black box warning from the FDA warning of risks for torsades de pointes associated with a single dose of 16 mg or a 24-hour total of 32 mg.[46] Each of the six patients had the same order, 4 mg of ondansetron every 8 hours, which is a maximum of 12 mg in 24 hours, significantly less than the black box warning. The other high-risk medication was haloperidol prescribed for one patient who was also receiving two intermediate-risk medications. For patients who are on immediate-risk medications, the presence of preexisting QTc prolongation or combination drug therapy including more than one intermediate-risk medication, increases the risk for the patient to develop torsades de pointes.[45] Four of seven patients received combination therapy, but only one patient had a preexisting slightly prolonged QTc.

Length of monitoring
The provider orders for telemetry specified duration of monitoring for either 24 or 48 hours. The mean gap of time between the predicted and actual length of monitoring was 43 hours and 10 minutes (**Table 4**). Thirteen patients were monitored for shorter time-periods than predicted (negative time); 78 patients were monitored longer than ordered (positive time). Of the 35 patients who had active telemetry orders when they changed levels of care, 22 were discharged from the hospital, six were taken to the operating room, four were transferred to the medical intensive care unit, and three were transferred to another unit.

Alarm Safety Survey Results

The survey was completed by 64 (60%) of eligible registered nurses from the study units. Most clinical nurses (43.3%; n = 29) had three or fewer years of experience, 28.4% (n = 19) had 3 to 6 years of experience, 11.9% (n = 8) had 6 to 11 years of experience, and 16.4% (n = 11) had greater than 11 years of experience. **Table 5** reports the descriptive statistics (means and standard deviations) for each of the 20 items on the HTF "Perceptions, Issues, Improvements, and Priorities of Healthcare

Table 4			
Predicted versus actual length of monitoring time			
	Negative Time	**Positive Time**	**Overall Time**
Mean	−13	58:16	43:10
Standard deviation	10:42	60:27	61:18
Range	−32:36 to −0:06	0:10–281:04	32:3–281:04

Time: hours:minutes.
  Negative time: the actual length of time on the monitor was less than predicted.
  Positive time: the actual length of time on the monitor was greater than predicted.

Table 5
Descriptive statistics for the HTF instrument by unit

	Medical Unit			Surgical Unit			
	n	Mean	Std. Dev	N	Mean	Std. Dev	Sig. *P* Value
1. Alarm sounds and/or visual displays should differentiate the priority of alarm	40	4.73	0.45	24	4.83	0.48	NS
2. Alarm sounds and/or visual displays should be distinct based on the parameter (eg, heart rate) or source (device type)	40	4.50	0.60	24	4.62	0.71	NS
3. Nuisance alarms occur frequently	40	4.32	0.94	24	4.29	0.91	NS
4. Nuisance alarms disrupt patient care	40	4.40	0.78	24	4.21	0.88	NS
5. Nuisance alarms reduce trust in alarms and cause caregivers to inappropriately turn alarms off at times other than setup or procedural events	40	4.25	0.78	24	4.21	0.93	NS
6. Properly setting alarm parameters and alerts is overly complex in existing devices	40	3.28	1.01	24	3.17	1.31	NS
7. Newer monitoring systems (eg, less than 3 y old) have solved most of the previous problems we experienced with clinical alarms	40	2.75	0.78	24	2.88	0.54	NS
8. The integration of clinical alarms into the Joint Commission patient safety measures, have reduced patient adverse events	40	3.53	0.75	24	3.37	0.71	NS
9. The alarms used on my floor/area of the hospital are adequate to alert staff of potential or actual changes in a patient's condition	40	3.70	0.76	24	3.71	1.08	NS
10. There have been frequent instances where alarms could not be heard and were missed	40	2.88	1.11	24	3.21	1.14	NS
11. Clinical staff is sensitive to alarms and responds quickly	40	3.63	0.93	24	3.17	1.13	NS

(continued on next page)

Table 5
(continued)

	Medical Unit			Surgical Unit			Sig. P Value
	n	Mean	Std. Dev	N	Mean	Std. Dev	
12. The medical devices used on my unit/floor all have distinct outputs (ie, sounds, repetition rates, visual displays) that allow users to identify the source of the alarm	40	3.53	0.88	24	3.58	1.02	NS
13. When several devices are used with a patient, it is confusing to determine which device is in an alarm condition	40	3.10	0.98	24	2.96	1.12	NS
14. Environmental background noise has interfered with alarm recognition	40	3.58	0.98	24	3.04	0.95	NS
15. Central alarm management staff responsible for receiving alarm messages and alerting appropriate staff is helpful	40	3.33	0.89	24	3.54	0.98	NS
16. Alarm integration and communication systems via pagers, cell phones, and other wireless devices are useful for improving alarms management and response	40	3.85	0.86	24	3.87	0.95	NS
17. Smart alarms (eg, where multiple parameters, rate of change of parameters, and signal quality, are automatically assessed in their entirety) would be effective to use for reducing false alarms	40	4.00	0.68	24	4.38	0.58	.029
18. Smart alarms (eg, where multiple parameters, rate of change of parameters, and signal quality, are automatically assessed in their entirety) would be effective to use for improving clinical response to important patient alarms	40	3.97	0.66	24	4.33	0.64	.036
19. Clinical policies and procedures regarding alarm management are effectively used in my facility	40	3.38	0.87	24	3.42	0.83	NS
20. There is a requirement in your institution to document that the alarms are set and are appropriate for each patient	40	4.20	0.56	24	3.83	0.92	NS

Pairwise comparisons performed with Mann–Whitney U tests.
Abbreviation: Std Dev, standard deviation.

Professionals" survey. There were no statistically significant differences between units on mean scores for all of the items, except for two items. Clinical nurses from the surgical unit scored significantly higher on items 17 and 18 related to the benefits of smart alarms. These items asked whether smart alarms would be effective to use for reducing false alarms or effective to use for improving clinical response to important patient alarms. Smart alarms use decision support from multiple parameters before generating an alarm, to improve the specificity of the alarm.

Nurses on both units strongly agreed or agreed that sounds or visual displays should differentiate the priority of the alarm (99.5%) and should be distinct based on the parameter or source (95.5%). Nurses also strongly agreed or agreed that nuisance alarms occur frequently (88.1%), disrupt patient care (83.6%), and reduce trust in alarms (80.6%) (**Table 6**). Nuisance alarms play a key role in alarm fatigue, and concerns about nuisance alarms reflected in survey responses corroborate findings generated from national samples. Nurses ranked the importance of nine alarm safety issues. Frequent false alarms were ranked as the most important alarm safety issue, which is congruent with results from the 2006 and 2011 national surveys (**Table 7**).[43]

DISCUSSION
Improve and Control

The results of this practice analysis and alarm survey were shared at a weekly unit-based clinical leadership, a forum for the discussion of unit quality and patient safety, and unit council, unit-based shared governance forum, meetings on each of the respective units targeted for this project using an A3 reporting tool. The A3 tool assimilates multiple aspects of a focused process plan that details the background of the issue, current conditions, goals and targets, an analysis of the issue, proposed countermeasures, a plan, and a follow-up plan.[47,48] Support was solicited for ongoing participation in the process improvement project to develop countermeasures to address overuse of telemetry and the issues identified on the alarm safety survey related to nuisance alarms.

Findings from this study led to consideration of actionable strategies to disseminate practice through the unit-based clinical leadership teams and patient safety committee. First, the electronic order set was reevaluated for potential exclusion of orders executed for telemetry that were not within accepted evidence-based standards. The subsequent updated AHA guidelines for telemetry published after this project was completed introduced new criteria to enhance the electronic order set for

Table 6
HTF survey: questions with greatest positive scores

Question	% Strongly Agree	% Agree	% Total
Alarm sounds and/or visual displays should differentiate the priority of alarm	76.12	23.39	99.51
Alarm sounds and/or visual displays should be distinct based on the parameter (eg, heart rate) or source (device type)	59.70	35.82	95.52
Nuisance alarms occur frequently	53.73	34.33	88.06
Nuisance alarms disrupt patient care	52.24	31.34	83.58
Nuisance alarms reduce trust in alarms and cause caregivers to inappropriately turn alarms off at times other than setup or procedural events	46.27	34.33	80.60

Table 7	
Rank order of alarm safety priorities (lower scores, higher priority)	
Alarm Safety Issue	**Score**
Frequent false alarms, which lead to reduced attention or response to alarms when they occur	3.45
Difficulty in hearing alarms when they occur	4.46
Difficulty in identifying the source of an alarm	4.76
Difficulty in understanding the priority of an alarm	4.88
Inadequate staff to respond to alarms as they occur	5.00
Difficulty in understanding the priority of an alarm	5.14
Noise competition from nonclinical alarms and pages	5.30
Difficulty in setting alarms properly	5.74
Lack of training on alarm systems	6.19

telemetry monitoring.[36] An order set based on the new guidelines addressed clinical decision processes regarding the use of telemetry for patients who do not meet a clinical indication for such monitoring. Additionally, the new AHA guidelines are likely to narrow the gap between the predicted and actual length of monitoring. The development of a nurse-driven telemetry discontinuation protocol is now part of the health system's strategic priority and is under development. This protocol holds promise for enabling nurses to evaluate the ongoing need for telemetry and make autonomous decisions to discontinue monitoring based on specified criteria. This impactful strategy may decrease the number of hours on telemetry, avoid the delivery of non-value-added care, and potentially represent substantial cost avoidance for the hospital. Engagement of all providers is essential to any efforts in updated order sets in the EMR and successfully executing a nurse-driven protocol for telemetry monitoring.

Our survey results demonstrate that nurses recognize nuisance alarms as a major alarm safety issue. The assessment of perceptions and practices related to alarm safety are critical to implementing measures to reduce unnecessary telemetry monitoring through evidence-based patient selection criteria for determining the need for such monitoring and adjustments to monitoring parameters to decrease nuisance alarms. Nurse practice leaders must be proactive in supporting ongoing surveillance of monitoring practices, optimizing policies and procedures to promote safe patient environments of care, and modifying behaviors related to alarm fatigue.

Project Limitations

The authors acknowledge limitations related to an observational analysis of practice. First, this study was conducted in a single academic medical center limiting the generalizability to other clinical settings. Second, data collection took place on two inpatient units with diverse medical and surgical patient populations. The model for telemetry monitoring involved nurse accountability for the interpreting telemetry monitoring information and responding to monitoring events. Other models for telemetry monitoring can include a monitor technician or a telemetry technician who assist nurses in surveillance and response to monitoring events affecting generalizability to patient care settings. Third, data were only collected over 28 days, which may not have been long enough to obtain a representative capture of practice patterns with telemetry. Fourth, assessments of congruence of the patient's clinical status with orders and evidence-based guidelines were based on documentation in the EMR, and as such, incomplete documentation was likely evident. Fifth, the scope of the process methodology for this project did not allow for the completion of the Improve and Control components of DMAIC. Data gathered from this project were shared with unit clinical nurses and nurse leaders to inform subsequent strategies to improve alarm management. Lastly, we did not survey physicians and APPs, and recognize that their perceptions and attitudes regarding telemetry monitoring are vital to understanding practice patterns associated with telemetry practices.

The response to our survey was robust with 60% of all eligible staff completing the survey. The information gained from the provider order analysis was helpful in understanding deviations in telemetry prescribing and duration from evidence-based practice guidelines. The measurement of the time gap between the anticipated and actual time on telemetry yielded greater transparency in the overuse of telemetry, which is associated with increased hospital costs and use of nursing staffing resources.

SUMMARY

Telemetry monitoring assesses clinical data that infrequently detect a change in patient status,[12,34] and therefore should be implemented according to evidence-based guidelines. Unnecessary or delayed use of telemetry may introduce nuisance alarms and noise into the clinical environment that distracts clinicians from focusing on important aspects of patient care. Telemetry can increase patient safety for cardiac or other health conditions as a noninvasive surveillance strategy when warranted, but it is not a surrogate for nurse interactions with patients to assess vital physiologic parameters. Distractions are a primary root cause for patient safety events, and the elimination of these distractions is essential to promoting safe practice environments. This study demonstrates the need to reevaluate telemetry practices to ensure that this type of monitoring aligns with the best available evidence and adds value to patient care. Nurses should participate in clinical decisions to determine those patients who can benefit from telemetry monitoring and the duration of monitoring. Moreover, nurses must establish individualized monitoring parameters to signal important clinical changes in a patient's status and troubleshoot problems that can reduce nuisance alarms and alarm fatigue.

REFERENCES

1. Purbaugh T. Alarm fatigue: a roadmap for mitigating the cacophony of beeps. Dimens Crit Care Nurs 2014;33(1):4–7.
2. Sendelbach S. Alarm fatigue. Nurs Clin North Am 2012;47(3):375–82.
3. Phillips J. Clinical alarms: complexity and common sense. Crit Care Nurs Clin North Am 2006;18(2):145–56.
4. Christensen M, Dodds A, Sauer J, et al. Alarm setting for the critically ill patient: a descriptive pilot survey of nurses' perceptions of current practice in an Australian regional critical care unit. Intensive Crit Care Nurs 2014;30(4):204–10.
5. Cvach M. Monitor alarm fatigue: an integrative review. Biomed Instrum Technol 2012;46(4):268–77.
6. Sendelbach S, Funk M. Alarm fatigue: a patient safety concern. AACN Adv Crit Care 2013;24(4):378–86.
7. Graham KC, Cvach M. Monitor alarm fatigue: standardizing use of physiological monitors and decreasing nuisance alarms. Am J Crit Care 2010;19(1):28–34.
8. Ryherd EE, Okcu S, Ackerman J, et al. Noise pollution in hospitals: impacts on staff. J Clin Outcomes Manag 2012;19(11):301–9.

9. The Joint Commission, Patient Safety Advisory Group. Medical device alarm safety in hospitals. Sentinel Event Alert Number 50. 2013. Available at: https://www.jointcommission.org/sea_issue_50/. Accessed July 4, 2018.

10. Blake N. The effect of alarm fatigue on the work environment. AACN Adv Crit Care 2014;25(1):18–9.

11. Welch J. Alarm fatigue hazards: the sirens are calling. JAMA 2012;307(15):1591–2.

12. Feder S, Funk M. Over-monitoring and alarm fatigue: for whom do the bells toll? Heart Lung 2013;42(6):395–6.

13. Görges M, Markewitz BA, Westenskow DR. Improving alarm performance in the medical intensive care unit using delays and clinical context. Anesth Analg 2009;108(5):1546–52.

14. Drew BJ, Califf RM, Funk M, et al. AHA scientific statement: practice standards for electrocardiographic monitoring in hospital settings: an American Heart Association scientific statement from the Councils on Cardiovascular Nursing, Clinical Cardiology, and Cardiovascular Disease in the Young: endorsed by the International Society of Computerized Electrocardiology and the American Association of Critical-Care Nurses. J Cardiovasc Nurs 2005;20(2):76–106.

15. Legge A. A review of the top 10 health technology hazards and how to minimise their risks. Nursing Times.net. 2009. Available at: http://www.nursingtimes.net/nursing-practice/clinical-zones/management/a-review-of-the-top-10-health-technology-hazards-and-how-to-minimise-their-risks/5005130.article. Accessed July 4, 2018.

16. Top 10 technology hazards for 2009. Health Devices 2008;37(11):343–50.

17. ECRI. ECRI Institute releases top 10 health technology hazards report for 2014. Health Devices 2013;42(11):1–16. Available at: https://www.ecri.org/Resources/Whitepapers_and_reports/2014_Top_10_Hazards_Executive_Brief.pdf. Accessed July 4, 2018.

18. Marion J. ECRI identifies top 10 health technology hazards for 2010. Healthcare IT News 2009. Available at: https://www.healthcareitnews.com/news/ecri-identifies-top-10-health-technology-hazards-2010#gs.CI3u7=8. Accessed July 4, 2018.

19. Schmidt B. ECRI Institute releases top 10 health technology hazards for 2011. Patient Safety and Quality in Healthcare; 2010. Available at: https://www.psqh.com/news/ecri-institute-releases-top-10-health-technology-hazards-for-2011/. Accessed July 4, 2018.

20. ECRI's top 10 health technology hazards for 2012. Newsl Biomed Saf Stand 2012;42(2):9–10.

21. Orlovsky C. The top health technology hazards for 2013. Healthcare News 2013. Available at: http://www.amnhealthcare.com/latest-healthcare-news/2147483683/1033/. Accessed July 4, 2018.

22. Medical Device Reporting. The Food and Drug Administration. 2014. Available at: http://www.fda.gov/medicaldevices/safety/reportaproblem/default.htm. Updated March 28, 2018. Accessed July 4, 2018.

23. Whalen DA, Covelle PM, Piepenbrink JC, et al. Novel approach to cardiac alarm management on telemetry units. J Cardiovasc Nurs 2014;29(5):E13–22.

24. The Joint Commission. Sentinel events policy and procedures. 2017. Available at: https://www.jointcommission.org/sentinel_event_policy_and_procedures/. Accessed July 7, 2018.

25. Benjamin EM, Klugman RA, Luckmann R, et al. Impact of cardiac telemetry on patient safety and cost. Am J Manag Care 2013;19(6):e225–32.

26. Dressler R, Dryer MM, Coletti C, et al. Altering overuse of cardiac telemetry in non-intensive care unit settings by hardwiring the use of the American Heart Association guidelines. JAMA Intern Med 2014;174(11):1852–4.
27. Henriques-Forsythe MN, Ivonye CC, Jamched U, et al. Is telemetry overused? Is it as helpful as thought? Cleve Clin J Med 2009;76(6):368–72.
28. Kanwar M, Fares R, Minnick S, et al. Inpatient cardiac telemetry monitoring: are we overdoing it? J Clin Outcomes Manag 2008;15(1):16–20.
29. Schull MJ, Redelmeier DA. Continuous electrocardiographic monitoring and cardiac arrest outcomes in 8,932 telemetry ward patients. Acad Emerg Med 2000; 7(6):647–52.
30. Bitan Y, Meyer J, Shinar D, et al. Nurses' reactions to alarms in a neonatal intensive care unit. Cogn Technol Work 2004;6(4):239–46.
31. Gazarian PK, Carrier N, Cohen R, et al. A description of nurses' decision-making in managing electrocardiographic monitor alarms. J Clin Nurs 2015;24(1–2): 151–9.
32. Gazarian PK. Nurses' response to frequency and types of electrocardiography alarms in a non-critical care setting: a descriptive study. Int J Nurs Stud 2014; 51(2):190–7.
33. Bulger J, Nickel W, Messler J, et al. Choosing wisely in adult hospital medicine: five opportunities for improved healthcare value. J Hosp Med 2013;8(9):486–92.
34. Kansara P, Jackson K, Dressler R, et al. Potential of missing life-threatening arrhythmias after limiting the use of cardiac telemetry. JAMA Intern Med 2015; 175(8):1416–8.
35. Cleverley K, Mousavi N, Stronger L, et al. The impact of telemetry on survival of in-hospital cardiac arrests in non-critical care patients. Resuscitation 2013;84(7): 878–82.
36. Sandau KE, Funk M, Auerbach A, et al. Update to practice standards for electrocardiographic monitoring in hospital settings: a scientific statement from the American Heart Association. Circulation 2017;136(19):e273–344.
37. Dhillon SK, Rachko M, Hanon S, et al. Telemetry monitoring guidelines for efficient and safe delivery of cardiac rhythm monitoring to noncritical hospital inpatients. Crit Pathw Cardiol 2009;8(3):125–6.
38. Gatien M, Perry JJ, Stiell IG, et al. A clinical decision rule to identify which chest pain patients can safely be removed from cardiac monitoring in the emergency department. Ann Emerg Med 2007;50(2):136–43.
39. Grossman SA, Shapiro NI, Mottley JL, et al. Is telemetry useful in evaluating chest pain patients in an observation unit? Intern Emerg Med 2011;6(6):543–6.
40. Leighton H, Kianfar H, Serynek S, et al. Effect of an electronic ordering system on adherence to the American College of Cardiology/American Heart Association guidelines for cardiac monitoring. Crit Pathw Cardiol 2013;12(1):6–8.
41. Pande PS, Neuman RP, Cavanagh RR. The six sigma way team fieldbook: an implementation guide for project improvement teams. New York: McGraw-Hill; 2002.
42. American Society for Quality. To DMAIC or not to DMAIC? 2012. Available at: http://asq.org/quality-progress/2012/11/back-to-basics/to-dmaic-or-not-to-dmaic. html. Accessed July 4, 2018.
43. Funk M, Clark JT, Bauld TJ, et al. Attitudes and practices related to clinical alarms. Am J Crit Care 2014;23(3):e9–18.
44. Drew BJ, Ackerman MJ, Funk M, et al. Prevention of torsades de pointes in hospital settings: a scientific statement from the American Heart Association and the

American College of Cardiology foundation. J Am Coll Cardiol 2010;55(9): 934–47.

45. AZCERT, Inc. Combined list of drugs that prolong QT and/or cause torsades de pointes (TDP). Credible Meds; 2018. Available at: https://crediblemeds.org/pdftemp/pdf/CombinedList.pdf. Accessed July 3, 2018.

46. Food and Drug Administration. New information regarding QT prolongation with ondansetron (Zofran). The Food and Drug Administration FDA Drug Safety Communication; 2012. Available at: http://www.fda.gov/Drugs/DrugSafety/ucm310190.htm. Accessed July 4, 2018.

47. Jimmerson C. Value stream mapping for healthcare made easy. New York: CRC Press; 2010.

48. The Lean Corner. (n.d.). Lean templates. Available at: http://theleancorner.com/free-templates/. Accessed July 7, 2018.

Impact of Nurse-Led Interprofessional Rounding on Patient Experience

Denise K. Gormley, PhD, RN[a], Amy J. Costanzo, PhD, RN-BC[b],*,
Jane Goetz, MSN, RN, NEA-BC[b], Jahmeel Israel, MS[a],
Jessica Hill-Clark, MBA, MA[a], Tracy Pritchard, PhD[a],
Katherine Staubach, MSN, MEd, RN, CPPS[b]

KEYWORDS

- Patient experience • Interprofessional • Interprofessional rounds
- Interprofessional collaborative practice • Nursing

KEY POINTS

- Patient experience, which includes satisfaction, quality, and safety, is an integral part of health care reform as medical costs rise and increase the financial risk for consumers.
- Interprofessional Collaborative Practice (IPCP) has been recommended to improve the issues of fragmented, poor-quality health care (Institute of Medicine, 2010).
- Nurse-led interprofessional bedside rounds is a patient-centered care model implemented to increase patient satisfaction and experience.
- IPCP through nurse-led interprofessional bedside rounds improves communication and collaboration between providers and with patients.
- Results of this quality improvement project demonstrate increased patient experience scores as measured by the Hospital Consumer Assessment of Healthcare Providers and Systems.

Declaration of Interest: The authors report no conflicts of interest. The authors alone are responsible for the content and writing of this article.

Financial Disclosure: This project was supported by the Health Resources and Services Administration (HRSA) of the US Department of Health and Human Services (HHS) under grant number UD7HP28546 and Nurse Education, Practice, Quality and Retention–Interprofessional Collaborative Practice for $1.2 million. This information or content and conclusions are those of the authors and should not be construed as the official position or policy of, nor should any endorsements be inferred by HRSA, HHS, or the US Government.

[a] University of Cincinnati College of Nursing, 3110 Vine Street, Cincinnati, OH 45219, USA;
[b] Nursing Administration, University of Cincinnati Medical Center, 234 Goodman Street, Cincinnati, OH 45219, USA
* Corresponding author.
E-mail address: amy.costanzo@uchealth.com

INTRODUCTION

Patient experience is a significant priority for health care organizations, impacting Medicare and Medicaid reimbursement, market share, and quality and safety.[1,2] Patient experience includes the interactions that patients have with the health care system, including care from physicians, nurses, and other health care professionals in hospitals.[3] Health care reform has an emphasis on improving the patient experience, including patient satisfaction and quality, and decreasing the per capita cost of health care.[4] Team-based care, in addition to interprofessional collaborative practice, has been identified as critical to reforming health care and achieving the Institute for Health Care Improvement's triple aim, which is as follows: (1) improving health care through patient satisfaction and quality; (2) improving population health; and (3) reducing the cost of health care per person.[5] A fourth aim, improving the work life of health care providers, was added to create the Quadruple Aim.[6] The gold standard for measuring patient experience is Hospital Consumer Assessment of Healthcare Providers and Systems (HCAHPS). HCAHPS measures aspects of the patient experience that include, but are not limited to, communication with caregivers, medication management, responsiveness of staff, and discharge readiness.[7] Although HCAHPS scores are used as a pay for performance metric, scores may also influence patients' and families' health care decisions.

One strategy to improve patient experience is rounding. Patient rounding involves intentional visits from nurses and physicians to monitor patient care and progress. There is a variety of types of rounds. Each type of rounds has its own unique definition, purpose, and process. One type of rounds is teaching rounds. Teaching rounds are medical education rounds led by chief residents or attending physicians and are used for informing clinical decision making and reviewing patient progress while role modeling for medical students and physician residents.[8,9] Another type of rounds is leader/administrative rounds, whereby leadership teams, consisting of directors, managers, and supervisors, round periodically to assess patient experience, assess patient and employee satisfaction, and engage employees in the workplace.[10] Hourly rounds include caregivers and patients and are intentionally focused on patient safety and care needs during a hospital shift.[11] Although similar to hourly rounds, nursing rounds are focused on patient assessments, patient safety, medication administration, and other nursing interventions.[2] Each of these types of rounds is siloed and fragmented from other professions. In addition, some of these types of rounds do not include the patient and the family in care planning. Rounds are often conducted in a central location, like a conference room, whereas others occur at the bedside or outside the patient room. For example, Brandt[12] and Nedfors and colleagues[13] reported that rounding generally occurs in profession-specific groups, indicating the infrequency of participation of other health professions, especially nurses.

Care of patients in the hospital involves patient management by several different professions and may include nurses, physicians, pharmacists, rehabilitation therapists, social workers, and dieticians.[14] Efficient communication among members of the health care team is essential for providing quality patient care.[15] The Interprofessional Education Collaborative (IPEC)[16] has set forth interprofessional core competencies that reflect the value of open communication and teamwork in delivering quality patient care. The IPEC core competencies are values/ethics, roles/responsibilities, interprofessional communication, and team and teamwork and were developed to better achieve the Triple Aim.[16] Nevertheless, little evidence of interprofessional team rounds that include more than 2 disciplines is found in the literature. When all professions are not collaborating effectively, a lack of teamwork and communication among health care teams creates a fragmented care system for patients.[13] Communication issues are consistently among the top 3 reported causes of patient harm in the United States.[17] Patient harm, due to ineffective communication among health care team members, may cause delays in patient care, need for higher levels of care, permanent harm, or death.[15,17]

PURPOSE

The purpose of this quality improvement (QI) project was to implement nurse-led interprofessional bedside rounds that aimed to decrease fragmentation and improve communication among providers, patients, and their families. This article describes the patient experience outcomes of this project. Nurse-led interprofessional bedside rounds were implemented with a surgical oncology team on a 24-bed surgical unit at a Midwestern, urban academic level I trauma center. For the purposes of this article, the authors defined interprofessional bedside rounding as 2 or more disciplines meeting together, with the patient, at the bedside to review the plan of care, determine priorities, and coordinate and facilitate a patient's progression from one point of care to the next.[18,19] This definition is adapted from Sen and colleagues[18] and Reimer and Herbener[19] to include the patient at the bedside. Health care professions that participated in nurse-led interprofessional bedside rounds were nursing, medicine, social work, pharmacy, rehabilitation therapy, and nutrition. An outcome examined as part of this QI project was patient experience because it specifically related to communication with care providers, communication about medications, and discharge readiness.

IMPLEMENTATION OF NURSE-LED INTERPROFESSIONAL BEDSIDE ROUNDING

The QI design for this project was the Plan-Do-Study-Act (PDSA) model. The Institute for Healthcare Improvement recommends the PDSA cycle for process improvement change.[20,21] Plan refers to development of the change; Do is the implementation of the plan; Study is the evaluation of the project; and Act means refine the plan-based evaluation.

The nurse-led interprofessional bedside rounding project was a joint effort between a college of nursing at a large, Midwestern university and an urban level 1 trauma center. This project was supported by the Health Resources and Services Administration of the US Department of Health and Human Services. Institutional Review Board approval was obtained before beginning the project.

Plan: Planning the Project

Planning for implementation of nurse-led interprofessional bedside rounds began with the development of a steering committee. The committee included the principal investigator, coprincipal investigator, hospital project consultants, and directors from the participating health professions (nursing, medicine, social work, pharmacy, rehabilitation therapy, and nutrition). The steering committee met quarterly for 6 months before implementation of bedside rounds and discussed implementation planning, orientation of participants, barriers and challenges, and the program evaluation methods. Steering committee members were tasked with orienting participating professionals before implementation of nurse-led interprofessional bedside rounds.

All steering committee professionals participated in the development of the nurse-led interprofessional bedside rounds standardized communication tool. The tool was designed to facilitate review of pertinent information about the last 24 hours of care and care plans for the next 24 hours. A standardized communication tool was used because it can increase the reliability, consistency, and timeliness of communication in collaborative teamwork among health professions.[22] Profession-specific care priorities were included in the tool. **Table 1** shows the standardized communication tool (see **Table 1**).

A key component of project planning was to prepare the nurses who would be leading and participating in the nurse-led interprofessional bedside rounds. To do this, a Bedside Nurse Leadership Development workshop was created to improve confidence and self-efficacy: 2 competencies that would be important to nurses' roles in leading and participating in nurse-led interprofessional bedside rounds. The Bedside Nurse Leadership Development workshop provided the opportunity for nurses to enhance leadership skills through active learning, didactic presentations, exploration of values, and role-playing. Role-play included time for nurses to practice facilitating and

---

Table 1
Standardized communication tool for bedside rounds

Charge nurse:
- Introduce patient to bedside rounds
- Ask permission to discuss in front of family/visitors if present

Bedside registered nurse:
- Update regarding last 24 h (mental status, vital signs, pertinent assessment, unanticipated events, intake and output)
- Pain
- Diet
- Safety
- Fall risk
- Isolation (type and precautions)
- Venous thromboembolism prophylaxis
- Mobility
- Compression boots
- Medications (ie, heparin, lovenox)
- Lines (central line, Foley, nasogastric, and similar)
- Infection concerns

Physician, Nurse Practitioner, Physician's Assistant: • Gives the team history of present illness • Active problems • Pertinent test results/consults	**Rehabilitation services:** • Strength and mobility • Progression plan
Dietary: • Current diet (tube feeds/total parenteral nutrition) • Caloric needs and calorie counts	**Respiratory therapy:** • Recommended treatment or therapy changes • Other respiratory concerns
Pharmacy: • Reconcile meds • Intravenous to oral conversion • Discuss discharge medications • Work with physicians to discontinue any unneeded medications • Drug levels	**Social work/case management:** • Status: outpatient, inpatient • Anticipated discharge date • Discharge disposition: home/facility/rehabilitation • Transportation • Are medications covered? • Hand held nebulizer, therapy, and durable medical equipment • Appointments to be scheduled

Charge nurse:
- Address goals for discharge date with patient
- What questions do you have for any members of the team

participating in nurse-led interprofessional bedside rounds. Scenarios were also provided to help nurses anticipate situations that might occur during rounds, for example, facilitating a long-winded clinician or a health professional absent from rounds.

Do: Implementation of Nurse-Led Interprofessional Bedside Rounds

Nurse-led interprofessional bedside rounds were implemented in January 2016 and continued through June 2018 on a surgical oncology unit at the partner hospital. The steps for nurse-led interprofessional bedside rounds are outlined as follows:

1. The rounding team met at a standing time and place each weekday.
2. The patient's bedside nurse provided a brief orientation to the patient and family to introduce rounds and offer the option to participate in care planning.
3. The charge nurse facilitated rounds by introducing the team to the patient and family and began the process of interprofessional rounds.
4. The bedside nurse began rounds with report of the patient's progress and concerns from the previous 24 hours using the standardized communication tool.
5. Medicine, pharmacy, social work, rehabilitation therapy, and nutrition provided their profession-specific report and patient goals, also using the standardized communication tool.
6. The patient and family were asked if they have questions.
7. The charge nurse provided a brief summary along with goals for the next 24 hours, including anticipated discharge date.
8. The patient communication board in the room was updated with the goals for the day and anticipated discharge date. Daily goals were an important communication element discussed with the team, patient, and family.

Study/Act: Evaluation of Rounding Process

During the first several months of implementation, members of the steering committee provided just-in-time coaching and debriefing of the interprofessional team. Coaching included requests for the team to use layman's terms in communicating with patients and families, time management during rounds, and use of the standardized tool. The nurse-led interprofessional bedside rounds process was modified over time using PDSA methodology and based on comments from patients and team members. Early during the implementation of nurse-led interprofessional bedside rounds, the standardized communication tool was modified based on feedback from the interprofessional team. For example, additional patient safety and quality indicators were added to the tool. Some of the feedback included the need for an onboarding orientation of new team members, order of reporting, and restructuring the order in which rounds occurred. Team members also recommended changing the time of rounds to better accommodate workflow and productivity.

Another way team members provided feedback was through formal focus groups led by 2 project evaluators. Providers who participated in nurse-led interprofessional bedside rounds were asked to reflect on their rounding experience. Audio recordings from the focus groups were transcribed, and any identifiers removed. Data were analyzed using conventional content analysis. Each focus group question was coded and summarized. Findings were shared with the steering committee to make recommended improvements to the nurse-led interprofessional bedside rounding process. The focus groups provided an opportunity for participants to provide open and honest feedback about the process in the event that they may be less comfortable sharing that during the in-person coaching or debriefing sessions. **Table 2** provides the codes and definitions derived from the focus groups.

Table 2
Focus group analysis

Code	Definition
1. Interprofessional collaboration/ communication prerounds	Interprofessional communication prerounding was described as occurring through 2 primary mechanisms: daily care conference and standard daily interaction. Care conference was described as a daily setting in which predominately nurses would convene at their own convenience in the conference room, although the other disciplines were welcome to attend, updates and changes on the patient were addressed during care conference. Care conference did not include the patient. Standard daily interactions, included going directly to the person or calling the person. The interviewees did describe that there were times for missed communication.
2. Interprofessional collaboration/ communication: postrounds	Interprofessional collaboration postrounds was described as a sure thing of connecting with the team during a planned meeting and knowing the plan. It is of note that participants consistently referred the patient as part of the process and increased patient and provider accountability.
3. The archetype of nurse-led bedside rounding	Bedside rounding was defined as a patient-centered coordination process to get everyone on the same page. It is a quick run assessment that includes the patient's voice as part of the team for accountability and allows team members to focus on what's important and patient satisfaction. However, this interdisciplinary communication mechanism to coordinate care where the nurse has control is different from traditional teaching rounds.
4. Reality of rounding	Participants frequently discussed that although the model of rounding was clear, protocol can be difficult to follow based on the reality of being a nurse on the unit. The reality of rounds included: the patient's voice can cause a deviation to the streamline of the rounding process, the stress of staying within the time limits with each round, the redundancy because the physician conducts their own rounds at a separate time, the limitations of the script, expectations are different for the nurses compared with other team members.
5. Training	Participants thought that the training they received was adequate. Participants described the process as making you remember important things to bring up for everybody to hear. Participants also noted the script has flaws and is unrealistic. There is no onboarding process for new RNs. Participants thought there were a lot of little glitches but thought they were prepared.
6. Likes	Participants like interprofessional rounds because it is efficient, gets everyone on the same page, and solidifies patient care plans. It was noted that the patient is a part of the team process and has a voice in holding the team accountable. Participants are focused, able to get answers and identify goals. They also like that the patient is involved but they are rushed. Participants like when every discipline involved is there and someone from the team is present to tell the patient the plan.

(continued on next page)

Code	Definition
Table 2 **(continued)**	
Code	**Definition**
7. Dislikes	Dislikes of interprofessional rounds centered on the effects on productivity standards and impacts on patient care because rounds were viewed as taking time away from other patients on that provider's service. Participants found the rounding process long and redundant with introductions. Participants described difficulty in balancing rounds within their workday, such as taking lunch, attending nursing grand rounds for CEs.
8. Changes in attitude and behavior	Participant's attitude and behavior changed to reflect patient-centered focus, emphasized use of plain language, focus on smaller things, and seeing the bigger picture, more prepared and better relationships. The impact of rounds allows team members not to miss as much as it relates to patient care. Not all changes in attitude and behavior were positive with feelings of bitterness that other disciplines are not held to the same accountability.
9. Perceptions of patient feedback	Feedback from patients was perceived as ambivalent, great, and positive and puts new patients at ease. Some patients refused rounds, but these were typically from long-term stay patients and were overwhelmed. Participants discussed that the patient's mood that day or personality can influence whether they want rounds.
10. Suggestions	Suggestions for improvement included better time management of rounds, elimination of the care conference, changing the time rounds are held, reestablishing the order in which patients are rounded on, defining the philosophy of rounds, revising the script, involving the bedside nurses with the project team, increasing feedback to the persons rounding.
11. Barriers to rounding	The barriers that emerged from the focus group included finding common time for all disciplines to meet, time constraint of the rounds, patient's voice, other patient needs, and inconsistent participation by all disciplines.

Study/Act: Evaluation of Patient Experience

Patient experience was measured by HCAHPS scores as an outcome of nurse-led interprofessional bedside rounds. HCAHPS was developed by the Agency for Healthcare Research and Quality[3] and the Centers for Medicare and Medicaid Services[7] to evaluate patients' experiences with hospital care. HCAHPS survey questions ask for patients' perceptions of care. This project specifically examined the questions related to communication of caregivers, communication about medications, and communication and coordination around discharge planning and readiness. Specific HCAHPS domains included in the evaluation of bedside rounds were: "Communication with Nurses," "Communication with Doctors," "Communication about Medicines," and "Discharge Information." HCAHPS data for the surgical oncology unit were analyzed for 2 years before, and almost 3 years after, implementation of rounds. Before scores and after scores were compared to establish the impact of nurse-led interprofessional bedside rounds on the patient experience.

RESULTS
Patient Experience

HCAHPS domain scores for patient experience for communication with nurses, communication with doctors, communication about medicines, and discharge information from calendar years 2014 and 2015 were compared with scores from calendar years 2016 and 2017. After nearly 3 years of implementation, all 4 of these domains in HCAHPS for the surgical oncology service increased.

Fig. 1 shows the comparison of the HCAHPS domain scores preimplementation and postimplementation of nurse-led interprofessional bedside rounds. The domain scores related to communication with doctor, communication with nurses, communication about medicines, and discharge readiness improved each year of the QI project over the previous 2 years preimplementation of rounds. The largest increases occurred for patient satisfaction with communication with nurses and communication about medicines with each having nearly 9.4 and 11.5 percentage point increases, respectively, from the initial baseline in calendar year 2014. **Fig. 2** demonstrates the comparison of the surgical oncology team with all unit patients, all hospital patients, and national benchmark scores through the 2017 calendar year.

Provider Experience with Implementation of Rounds

Health care providers who participated in nurse-led interprofessional bedside rounds were invited to participate in focus groups to share what interprofessional

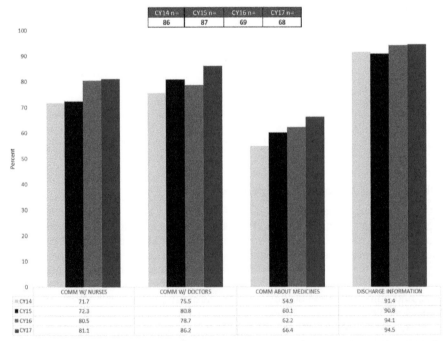

	CY14 n=	CY15 n=	CY16 n=	CY17 n=
	86	87	69	68

	COMM W/ NURSES	COMM W/ DOCTORS	COMM ABOUT MEDICINES	DISCHARGE INFORMATION
CY14	71.7	75.5	54.9	91.4
CY15	72.3	80.8	60.1	90.8
CY16	80.5	78.7	62.2	94.1
CY17	81.1	86.2	66.4	94.5

Fig. 1. HCAHPS score comparison from 2014 to 2017 on a surgical oncology unit. Scores for the domains of communication (comm) with nurses, communication with doctors, communication about medicines, and discharge information are shown as total percent satisfaction from calendar years (CY) 2014 to 2017. CY14-15 is preimplementation of nurse-led interprofessional bedside rounds.

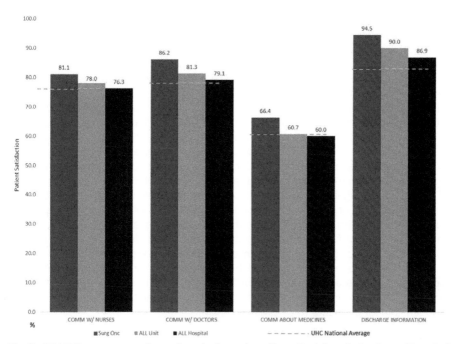

Fig. 2. HCAPHS score comparison of surgical oncology (Surg Onc), hospital unit, and hospital overall for calendar year (CY) 2017. Patient satisfaction with communication (comm) with nurses, communication with doctors, communication about medicines, and discharge information is presented by surgical oncology, all unit, and all hospital. The national average benchmarks for each of these domains are presented as a dashed line.

collaborative practice looked like preimplementation and postimplementation of rounds, discuss how rounds were really carried out as compared with the formal understanding, and provide feedback on the training and barriers to implementation, as well as provide suggestions for improvement. Six focus groups were conducted with a total of 29 providers who participated in nurse-led interprofessional bedside rounds.

Table 2 shows the codes that were derived from the focus group questionnaire and summarized participant feedback. Key findings from the focus groups was the transformation of interprofessional collaboration on the unit, the realities of doing interprofessional rounding, importance of training, and suggestions based on positive and negative constructive feedback. The most significant change in the way interprofessional collaborative practice was conducted on the unit was the inclusion of the patient as part of the care team. Having the rounds at the bedside and intentional acknowledgment of the patient as part of the team permitted a voice for the patient that was not included in interprofessional collaborative practice before rounding.

DISCUSSION

The surgical oncology rounding team that participated in nurse-led interprofessional bedside rounds exceeded patient experience benchmarks in all 4 of the targeted domains. The largest difference in patient experience between the surgical oncology unit and all unit patients was for communication about medicines, whereas the largest differences in patient satisfaction between the surgical oncology unit and the entire hospital were for communication with doctors and discharge information.

Although patient experience is a top priority at the hospital with many initiatives implemented over the years of this project to improve patient experience, **Figs. 1** and **2** demonstrate the higher scores obtained on the surgical oncology service through interprofessional bedside rounds over the scores from the remainder of the hospital. In each of the domains, the surgical oncology service surpassed the unit, hospital, and national benchmark scores.

This project collected data from a validated tool to evaluate the impact of patient experience. However, there is a lack of evidence in the literature on how interprofessional rounds correlate to patient experience or HCAHPS data. This QI project suggests a positive connection between nurse-led interprofessional bedside rounds and the patient experience metrics of "Communication with Nurses," "Communication with Doctors," "Communication about Medicines," and "Discharge Information."

Despite having significant planning and training for implementing and conducting rounds, the realities of providing patient care could at times interfere with the rounding process. Such realities included keeping the rounding process confined to a restricted time limit, limitations of the standardized communication tool, differences in staff expectations based on discipline, and the dynamics of inclusion of the patient voice in rounding.

Overwhelmingly providers expressed the benefits of the nurse-led interprofessional bedside rounds. Some recommendations for improvement included strategies for better managing time during rounds as well as changing the start time of rounds to make it more feasible for providers to be present on time.

SUMMARY

Nurse-led interprofessional bedside rounds was a QI project that is not generalizable; however, the nurse-led interprofessional bedside rounds process can be replicated in similar organizations. Other patient experience initiatives were implemented within the hospital during the implementation phase of nurse-led interprofessional bedside rounds. Nonetheless, the HCAHPS domain scores for the surgical oncology team showed greater improvement than the overall unit scores where the project occurred as well as in the other units in the organization.

Challenges arose during the planning and implementation of the nurse-led interprofessional bedside rounds project. For example, ongoing orientation of new staff to the project was not initially planned. The ideal time for all professions to round was not anticipated. The nurse-led interprofessional bedside rounds were a change from the traditional teaching and conference room rounds that previously occurred on the surgical oncology service. Alterations in workflow and conventional thinking take time and facilitation to establish workload expectations and direct caregiver stakeholder buy-in. Finally, navigation of diverse communication styles toward common interprofessional patient-centric communication was needed.

Recommendations to alleviate these challenges are as follows:

- Include participating professions in planning stages and use collaborative decision making with all professions;
- Continual facilitation of nurse-led interprofessional bedside rounds by the project team;
- Role modeling and coaching of nurse-led interprofessional bedside rounds behaviors from team leaders;
- Development of an orientation process for new staff to the nurse-led interprofessional bedside rounds project;
- Ongoing meetings with key stakeholders in the project to communicate successes and discuss barriers.

The nurse-led interprofessional bedside rounds QI project findings demonstrate a significant impact on patient experience as indicated in HCAHPS domain scores of "Communication with Nurses," "Communication with Doctors," "Communication about Medications," and "Discharge Information." This nurse-led interprofessional bedside rounds project is now in the sustainability phase. Much of the responsibility to maintain nurse-led interprofessional bedside rounds has been transitioned from the project team to the unit leadership team. Quarterly committee meetings with key stakeholders continue for evaluating the project and addressing ongoing challenges and barriers. The role of facilitation and coaching to establish and maintain the success of nurse-led interprofessional bedside rounds cannot be underestimated.

Patient experience is important to the patient and family as well as health care systems. Improved patient experience influences quality, safety, and reimbursement and decreases avoidable suffering.[15,17] This project demonstrated that nurse-led interprofessional bedside rounds that include multiple professions can improve communication between providers, patients, and families. This improved communication decreases fragmented care through all professions working toward the same patient goals.

REFERENCES

1. Berkowitz B. The patient experience and patient satisfaction: measurement of a complex dynamic. Online J Issues Nurs 2016;21(1):1.
2. Blakley D, Kroth M, Gregson J. The impact of nurse rounding on patient satisfaction in a medical-surgical hospital unit. Medsurg Nurs 2011;20(6):327–32. Available at: https://www.ncbi.nlm.nih.gov/pubmed/22409118.
3. Agency for Healthcare Research and Quality. What is patient experience? Agency for Healthcare Research and Quality, Rockville, MD. Available at: http://www.ahrq.gov/cahps/about-cahps/patient-experience/index.html. Accessed November 25, 2018.
4. Berwick DM, Nolan TW, Whittington J. The triple aim: care, health, and cost. Health Aff (Milwood) 2008;27:759–69.
5. Institute for Healthcare Improvement (IHI). Triple aim. Available at: http://www.ihi.org/Engage/Initiatives/TripleAim/Pages/default.aspx. Accessed March 9, 2018.
6. Sikka R, Morath JM, Leape L. The quadruple aim: care, health, cost and meaning in work. BMJ Qual Saf 2015;24(10):608–10.
7. The Centers for Medicare & Medicaid Services (CMS). Hospital CAHPS (HCAHPS) fact sheet. 2005. Available at: https://www.cms.gov/Medicare/Quality-Initiatives-Patient-Assessment-Instruments/HospitalQualityInits/Downloads/HospitalHCAHPSFactSheet.pdf. Accessed April 18, 2018.
8. Abdool MA, Bradley D. Twelve tips to improve medical teaching rounds. Med Teach 2013;35(11):895–9.
9. Cruess SR, Cruess RL, Steinert Y. Role modeling – making the most of a powerful teaching strategy. BMJ 2008;336(7646):718–21.
10. Winter M, Tjiong L. HCAHPS series part 2: does purposeful leader rounding make a difference? J Nurs Manag 2015;46(2):26–32.
11. Halm MA. Hourly rounds: what does the evidence indicate? Am J Crit Care 2009;18:581–4.
12. Brandt B. Interprofessional education and collaborative practice: welcome to the "new" forty-year-old field. The Advisor Online. 2015. Available at: http://www.naahp.org/publications/TheAdvisorOnline/Vol35No1/35-1-02.aspx. Accessed November 25, 2018.

13. Nedfors K, Borg C, Fagerstrom C. Communication with physicians in hospital rounds: an interview with nurses. Nord J Nurs Res 2015;36(3):122–7.
14. Sullivan M, Kiovsky R, Mason D, et al. Interprofessional collaboration and education. Am J Nurs 2015;115:47–54.
15. Cornell P, Townsend-Gervis M, Vardaman JM, et al. Improving situation awareness and patient outcomes through interdisciplinary rounding and structured communication. J Nurs Adm 2014;44(3):164–9.
16. Interprofessional Education Collaborative. Core competencies for interprofessional collaborative practice: 2016 update. Washington, DC: Interprofessional Education Collaborative; 2016.
17. The Joint Commission. Sentinel event alert 58: inadequate handoff communication. Oak Brook (IL): Joint Commission Resources; 2017.
18. Sen A, Xiao Y, Lee SA, et al. Daily multidisciplinary discharge rounds in a trauma center: a little time, well spent. J Trauma 2009;66(3):880–7.
19. Reimer N, Herbener L. Round and round we go: rounding strategies to impact exemplary professional practice. Clin J Oncol Nurs 2014;18(6):654–60.
20. Institute for healthcare improvement. Available at: http://www.ihi.org/resources/Pages/HowtoImprove/default.aspx. Accessed November 25, 2018.
21. Associates in process improvement. Available at: http://www.apiweb.org/. Accessed November 25, 2018.
22. Gurses AP, Xiao Y. A systematic review of the literature on multidisciplinary rounds to design information technology. J Am Med Inform Assoc 2006;13(3):267–76.

Reducing Pressure Injuries in the Pediatric Intensive Care Unit

Kristin A. Cummins, DNP, RN[a],*, Richard Watters, PhD, RN[b],
Treasa 'Susie' Leming-Lee, DNP, MSN, RN[c]

KEYWORDS

- Pressure injuries • Pressure ulcers • Pediatrics • Wounds • Skin integrity

KEY POINTS

- PICU nurses lack knowledge of pediatric pressure injury risk factors and causation.
- Nurse leaders must ensure PICU nurses remain up to date on evidence-based pressure injury prevention strategies.
- Pressure injuries are reduced by leveraging technology to link risk assessment tools with evidence-based prevention strategies.

Nationally, 2.5 million patients are affected by pressure injuries every year and it is estimated nearly 60,000 patients die each year from hospital-acquired pressure injury complications.[1] Research demonstrates most pressure injuries are preventable, therefore lives are saved by implementing and adhering to evidence-based pressure injury prevention strategies.[2] A pressure injury is defined as "localized tissue damage to the skin and underlying soft tissue usually over a bony prominence or related to a medical or other device."[3(px)] Research has found patients with pressure injuries are at an increased risk of infection, experience pain from the pressure injuries, and stay in the hospital longer than patients without pressure injuries.[4,5] With the recent focus on decreasing patient harm in hospital settings following the Institute of Medicine's landmark report To Err is Human,[6] The Joint Commission and the Institute for Healthcare Improvement have called attention to the importance of pressure injury prevention in health care facilities.[7,8]

Disclosure Statement: No disclosures.
[a] Quality and Safety Department, Riley Hospital for Children at Indiana University Health, 705 Riley Hospital Drive, Suite RI 2962, Indianapolis, IN 46202, USA; [b] Vanderbilt University School of Nursing, 461 21st Avenue South, 220 Godchaux Hall, Nashville, TN 37240, USA; [c] Vanderbilt University School of Nursing, 461 21st Avenue South, 216 Godchaux Hall, Nashville, TN 37240, USA
* Corresponding author.
E-mail address: Kcummin1@iuhealth.org

Although effective, evidence-based pressure injury prevention strategies have been identified in the adult population, these prevention strategies have not been proven effective in the pediatric population.[4,9] Pediatric intensive care unit (PICU) patients are at an increased risk of developing pressure injuries because of their unstable hemodynamic status and the multitude of invasive treatments and procedures they undergo.[10] The PICU is a technology-rich environment. Patients in the PICU often require a multitude of medical devices to support aggressive treatment requirements.[4] PICU patients often have ventilation needs, poor perfusion, and require inotropic support.[4,10] Additionally, PICU patients often are not turned routinely because of their fragile hemodynamic status.[10] Furthermore, hospitalized pediatric patients have a limited ability to communicate discomfort, pain, or the need to be repositioned.[11] With the incidence of pressure injuries in PICU being 27%, it is imperative evidence-based pediatric pressure injury prevention strategies are identified and evaluated.[4]

AIM STATEMENT

The aim of this quality improvement project was to implement evidence-based pediatric pressure injury prevention strategies to decrease the incidence of pressure injuries by reducing the rate from 8% to 6% in the PICU at a children's hospital in a large metropolitan city during a 6-week time period. The objectives were:

1. To deliver an education session on risk factors for pediatric pressure injuries and evidence-based prevention strategies to PICU nurses.
2. To educate PICU nurses on the importance of turning patients every 2 hours to increase compliance with provider orders.
3. To implement an electronic trigger in the electronic health record by collaborating with PICU providers, dieticians, and clinical informatics to automate the ordering of nutrition consultations for patient with Braden Q scores of 16 or less.

Conceptual Framework

The IOWA Model of Evidence-Based Practice to Promote Quality Care was used as the conceptual framework to guide the quality improvement project.[12] The IOWA Model of Evidence-Based Practice to Promote Quality Care is widely used by nurses to make clinical practice decisions to impact quality outcomes. The model is unique in that it allows for the evidence to be individualized to the specific practice setting in which the evidence is being implemented.[13] The model is seen in **Fig. 1**.

Literature Review

The authors conducted an integrative review of the literature on September 19, 2016, and October 17, 2016, to identify effective pediatric pressure injury prevention strategies. Six pediatric pressure injury prevention interventions appeared consistently across several studies: (1) ensuring proper support surfaces for patients, (2) turning patients frequently, (3) ensuring proper nutrition for patients, (4) managing moisture for patients, (5) conducting routine skin assessments, and (6) the use of skin champions on units. All six intervention strategies were shown to reduce pressure injury incidence or prevalence throughout the studies.[10,14–18]

Although the literature review resulted in the finding of six evidence-based pediatric pressure injury prevention strategies, three of the six specific interventions were eliminated after considering the current state of practice in the PICU at the hospital and the timeline for this quality improvement project. This quality improvement project

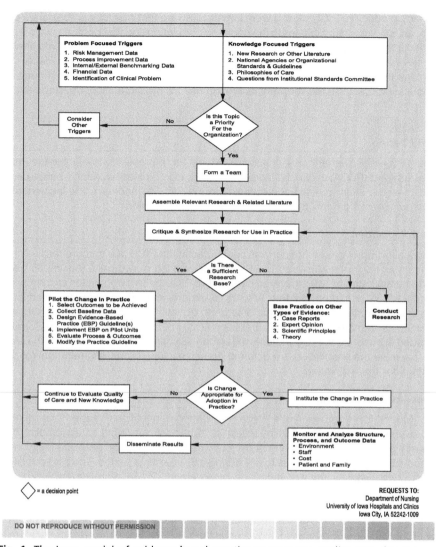

Problem Focused Triggers
1. Risk Management Data
2. Process Improvement Data
3. Internal/External Benchmarking Data
4. Financial Data
5. Identification of Clinical Problem

Knowledge Focused Triggers
1. New Research or Other Literature
2. National Agencies or Organizational Standards & Guidelines
3. Philosophies of Care
4. Questions from Institutional Standards Committee

Is this Topic a Priority For the Organization?

Consider Other Triggers — No

Yes

Form a Team

Assemble Relevant Research & Related Literature

Critique & Synthesize Research for Use in Practice

Is There a Sufficient Research Base?

Yes — Pilot the Change in Practice
1. Select Outcomes to be Achieved
2. Collect Baseline Data
3. Design Evidence-Based Practice (EBP) Guideline(s)
4. Implement EBP on Pilot Units
5. Evaluate Process & Outcomes
6. Modify the Practice Guideline

No — Base Practice on Other Types of Evidence:
1. Case Reports
2. Expert Opinion
3. Scientific Principles
4. Theory

Conduct Research

Is Change Appropriate for Adoption in Practice?

Continue to Evaluate Quality of Care and New Knowledge — No

Yes — Institute the Change in Practice

Monitor and Analyze Structure, Process, and Outcome Data
• Environment
• Staff
• Cost
• Patient and Family

Disseminate Results

◇ = a decision point

REQUESTS TO:
Department of Nursing
University of Iowa Hospitals and Clinics
Iowa City, IA 52242-1009

Fig. 1. The Iowa model of evidence-based practice to promote quality care. (*From* Iowa Model Collaboration. Iowa Model of evidence-based practice: Revisions and validation. Worldviews on Evidence-Based Nursing 2017;14(3):175–82; with permission.)

focused on increasing nursing compliance with turning PICU patients every 2 hours and instituting the routine ordering of nutrition consultations on all PICU patients with a Braden Q Scale risk score less than 16. The Braden Q Scale is a validated and reliable tool used to predict pediatric pressure injury risk.[19] A Braden Q Scale score of 16 or lower means the patient is at risk for developing a pressure injury.[19]

Additionally, an education session was delivered to the PICU nurses on medical devices being the primary cause of pressure injuries in pediatrics and the role of nutrition in preventing pressure injuries. These interventions were chosen primarily because 79% of the PICU pressure injuries are medical device related and 21% are immobility related. In addition, PICU nurses were largely unaware that medical devices are a primary cause of pressure injuries in the pediatric population and that nutrition plays such a critical role in decreasing susceptibility to pressure injuries in these patients. It was necessary to increase PICU nurses' knowledge of pediatric pressure injury causes to increase their compliance with turning patients every 2 hours and ensuring nutrition consultations are ordered for patients at high risk for pressure injury development.

METHODS
Study Design

This quality improvement project used the Model for Improvement including the Plan-Do-Study-Act (PDSA) cycle of change framework to implement evidence-based pediatric pressure injury prevention strategies in the PICU to decrease the incidence of pressure ulcers from 8% to 6% during a 6-week time period.[20]

Study Population

This quality improvement project was conducted in the PICU at a comprehensive children's hospital in the Midwest. The PICU is comprised of two units totaling 36 beds with a nursing staff of 112 registered nurses. The PICU patient population is comprised of critically ill or injured children who have experienced trauma, severe infections, congenital anomalies, immunologic disorders, or have undergone extensive surgery. All patients admitted to the PICU between May 7, 2017, and June 30, 2017, were included in the project. PICU patients older than 18 years were excluded from the project, because the hospital uses a different pressure injury risk assessment tool for patients older than 18 years.

Model for Improvement

The Model for Improvement's three foundational questions guided the quality improvement project. The first question is, "what are we trying to accomplish?"[20] The aim of the quality improvement project was to decrease the pressure injury incidence rate in the PICU from 8% to 6% during a 6-week time period. The next question is, "how will we know that a change is an improvement?"[20] An improvement was noted after implementing the evidence-based pressure injury prevention strategies resulted in a decrease in the incidence rate of pressure injuries in the PICU. Finally, "what changes can we make that will result in improvement?"[20] The changes used in this quality improvement project included educating PICU nurses on pressure injury risk factors and prevention strategies, increasing compliance with turning patients per physician order, and implementing an electronic trigger in the electronic health record to automate the ordering of nutrition consultations for patients with Braden Q scores of 16 or less.

Plan-do-study-act cycle

A PDSA cycle of change was used to implement the following three evidence-based pressure injury prevention strategies: (1) educating PICU nurses on risk factors for pediatric pressure injuries and prevention strategies, (2) turning PICU patients every 2 hours, and (3) ordering nutrition consultations on all patients with a Braden Q score less than 16. Several multidisciplinary groups were involved in the quality improvement project including the hospital executive team, clinical informatics, nursing education, nutrition support team, quality and safety leaders, and the PICU patient care team. The PICU patient care team roles that were involved included physicians, nurse practitioners, dieticians, nursing leaders, educators, and staff nurses.

Plan

The quality improvement project plan was vetted to the various multidisciplinary groups during January and February 2017. The project leader collaborated with the medical director of quality and safety to coordinate a series of meetings with key stakeholders to obtain their support and engagement for the quality improvement project. The chief nursing officer and chief medical officer were asked to support the quality improvement project by reinforcing the importance of the project to their direct reports who work in the PICU.

Education PICU nursing leaders asked all PICU nurses to complete pressure injury education during the project. The project leader developed the content for the pressure injury education using the literature review findings and collaborating with the hospital's wound and skin clinical nurse specialist. The pressure injury education content covered risk factors for pediatric pressure injuries, reinforced proper pressure injury documentation, and highlighted the importance of turning patients every 2 hours and obtaining nutrition consultations on patients with a Braden Q score less than 16.

Turning PICU nursing leaders planned to reinforce the importance of turning PICU patients every 2 hours by communicating with PICU staff nurses during daily rounding, at staff meetings, and via e-mail communication during the quality improvement project. The project leader developed a process for tracking daily turning compliance during the project by using the turning compliance audit tool. The project leader planned to request the PICU clinical nurse specialist follow-up on any PICU patients not being turned every 2 hours during the quality improvement project to identify and mitigate barriers to turning.

Nutrition The project leader obtained support from PICU providers and dieticians to complete nutrition consultations on PICU patients with a Braden Q score less than 16 and collaborate to develop a plan to optimize nutrition in PICU patients during the quality improvement project. The hospital's nutrition support team agreed to participate in the quality improvement project to provide expertise to the PICU providers and dieticians regarding how to optimize nutrition in medically complex children. The clinical informatics team committed to developing a trigger in the electronic medical record to automatically order a nutrition consultation on all patients with a Braden Q score less than 16.

Do

Institutional review board approval was obtained from Vanderbilt University on April 25, 2017, and Indiana University on May 18, 2017. The quality improvement project changes were implemented on May 21, 2017, through June 30, 2017 (**Fig. 2**). An email

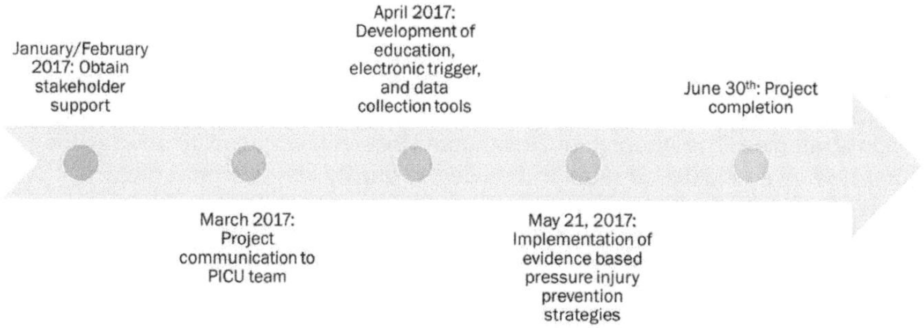

January/February 2017: Obtain stakeholder support

April 2017: Development of education, electronic trigger, and data collection tools

June 30th: Project completion

March 2017: Project communication to PICU team

May 21, 2017: Implementation of evidence based pressure injury prevention strategies

Fig. 2. Project plan timeline.

communication was sent to PICU nursing staff on May 21st reinforcing the importance of turning all patients every 2 hours and ensuring all patients with a Braden Q score less than 16 have nutrition consultations ordered. The project leader and the medical director of quality and safety rounded weekly on PICU to assess the quality improvement project's progress throughout the project's 6-week timeline.

Education The nursing education director partnered with the project leader to develop a pretest and posttest for the pressure injury education. These tests were used to assess for pressure injury knowledge improvement in PICU nurses before and following the delivery of the pediatric pressure injury education session. Nurses were asked to put their three initials at the top of the completed test to allow for comprehensive pretest and posttest data analysis. The education session was delivered electronically via video recording rather than in person as originally planned per PICU nursing leadership advisement. PICU nurses were asked to watch the video and complete the knowledge assessment posttest.

Turning The project leader tracked daily PICU patient turning compliance throughout the quality improvement project to assess for a change in compliance. The project leader collected turning data via chart reviews on a daily basis. Turning compliance rates were disseminated to the project team on a weekly basis.

Nutrition On June 20, 2017, the electronic trigger automating the ordering of nutrition consultations for patients with a Braden Q score of 16 or less was implemented in the PICU. Dieticians now receive a nutrition consultation order anytime a nurse completes a Braden Q scale risk assessment on a patient and scores the patient at 16 or less. The dieticians use the order to alert them to account for the patient's pressure injury risk in their nutrition recommendations to the PICU medical team. The project leader tracked nutrition consultation compliance to assess for a change in nutrition consultation ordering in PICU patients with a Braden Q score of 16 or less throughout the project. The project leader used electronic medical record reports to complete the tool.

Pressure injury incidence rate The project leader was notified of pressure injuries on PICU during the daily quality and safety team huddle at the hospital. The PICU clinical nurse specialist provided the project leader with information regarding the cause of the pressure injury and whether appropriate prevention strategies were in place. Electronic health record reports were used by the project leader to obtain the number of PICU admissions every week to determine the weekly pressure injury incidence rate. The project leader tracked weekly pressure injury incidence in the PICU throughout the quality improvement project.

Study

The aim of the quality improvement project was to reduce the incidence of pressure injuries in the PICU, therefore the primary outcome measure was pressure injury incidence. The project leader analyzed the pressure injury incidence rate in the PICU before, during, and after the implementation of evidence-based pressure injury prevention strategies. The Agency for Healthcare Research and Quality advises the use of pressure injury incidence rates to be used in quality improvement projects.[21] The project leader calculated pressure injury incidence rates weekly by dividing the number of patients who developed a pressure injury in the PICU within a week by the number of all patients admitted to the PICU during the same week. The project leader also calculated the monthly pressure injury incidence rate for the PICU throughout the quality improvement project.

Turning compliance and nutrition consultation compliance were the process measures contributing to the decrease in the pressure injury incidence rate in the PICU. The project leader analyzed the turning compliance data at the completion of the project to determine whether an increase in turning compliance occurred as a result of the quality improvement project. Nutrition consultation compliance data were analyzed at the end of the project to determine whether the percentage of nutrition consultations on high-pressure injury risk patients increased as a result of the quality improvement project.

PICU nurses' knowledge of pediatric pressure injury causes and prevention strategies was also an outcome measure for the quality improvement project and was assessed by the completion of pressure injury pretests and posttests. The pretests and posttests provided the project leader with the necessary data to conduct a paired *t* test to assess whether PICU nurses' knowledge of pressure injury causes and prevention strategies improved following the education. The quality improvement project interventions and corresponding data collections tools and measures are shown in **Table 1**.

Act

According to IOWA Model of Evidence-Based Practice to Promote Quality Care, the project team must evaluate whether changes that were piloted during the PDSA cycle should be implemented into practice.[12] The project team will decide to fully adopt and implement the pediatric pressure injury prevention strategies in the PICU if the pressure injury incidence rate decreases and sustains for 90 days after the completion of the quality improvement project. The project team will collaborate with the hospital's quality and safety leadership team to determine whether to spread the pediatric pressure injury prevention strategies across the hospital following the completion of the quality improvement project.

DATA ANALYSIS

Turning compliance and nutrition consultation compliance were compared preimplementation and postimplementation of evidence-based pressure injury prevention strategies to determine whether an improvement occurred. Weekly pressure injury incidence rates were analyzed during the quality improvement project to determine whether the evidence-based pressure injury prevention strategies decreased the incidence of pressure injuries in the PICU. Pressure injury knowledge assessment pretests and posttests were analyzed by paired *t* tests to determine whether the education provided to PICU nurses was effective. Excel was the software used for data analysis.

RESULTS
Pretest and Posttest

The PICU pressure injury education assessment pretest was completed by 51 PICU nurses and the posttest was completed by 29 PICU nurses (**Table 2**). PICU nurse demographics were collected on the pressure injury knowledge assessment posttest. Twenty-four PICU nurses completed the demographics section. Thirty-seven percent of the PICU nurses had zero to 2 years of experience as a pediatric nurse, 33% had between 2 and 7 years of experience, and 29% had more than 7 years' experience. Most (92%) of the PICU nurses worked full time with 58% working nightshift and 42% working dayshift.

Table 1
Quality improvement project interventions, data collection tools, and measures

Intervention	Methodology	Process Measure	Data Collection Tool	Outcome Measure
PICU nursing pressure injury education	Project leader delivered formal education to PICU nursing team on medical devices being a causative factor in pediatric pressure injuries and the role of nutrition in preventing pressure injuries	Percent of PICU nurses completing pressure injury education (number of PICU nurses who completed pressure injury education/ number of PICU nurses)	Pressure injury pretests and posttests	Paired t test to compare pretest and posttest means for PICU nurses to assess knowledge improvement following education
Turn PICU patients every 2 h	Nursing leadership reinforcement of need to turn patients every 2 h; daily compliance report to PICU nurses	Daily PICU patient turning compliance (number of PICU patients turned every 2 h/number of PICU patients)	Turning compliance audit tool	PICU pressure injury incidence
Ordering nutrition consultations on all PICU patients with a Braden Q score <16	Instituted electronic medical record trigger to order a nutrition consultation for all patients with a Braden Q score <16	% of PICU patients with a Braden Q score <16 with a nutrition consultation ordered	Daily electronic report of PICU patients with a Braden Q score <16 compared with a daily report of PICU patients with nutrition consultations ordered	PICU pressure injury incidence

The average score on the PICU pressure injury education assessment pretest was 61.6%. PICU nurses lacked knowledge on pressure injury causation (13.7%), pediatric pressure injury causation (29.4%), pediatric pressure injury risk factors (3.9%), patient outcomes associated with pressure injuries (23.5%), pediatric pressure injury occurrence time frame (39.2%), and Braden Q scale risk assessment (2%). The average score on the PICU pressure injury knowledge assessment posttest was 79.5%. Twenty-nine PICU nurses completed pretests and posttests to allow for paired t test analysis (**Table 3**). PICU nurses demonstrated a significant increase in knowledge following the pressure injury education session in the following areas: pressure injury causation ($t = 5.07$, $df = 28$; $P<.05$), pediatric pressure injury causation ($t = 3.37$, $df = 28$; $P<.05$), pediatric pressure injury risk factors ($t = 7.26$, $df = 28$; $P<.05$), patient outcomes associated with pressure injuries ($t = 2.38$, $df = 28$; $P<.05$), pressure injury prevalence reporting ($t = 2.19$, $df = 28$; $P<.05$), pressure injury location on small

Table 2		
PICU nursing staff knowledge assessment pre and post pressure injury education		
	Preintervention **(n = 51)**	**Postintervention** **(n = 29)**
Assessment Questions		
Causation	7 (13.7%)	16 (55.2%)
Pediatric causation	15 (29.4%)	14 (48.3%)
Risk factors	2 (3.9%)	16 (55.2%)
Outcomes	12 (23.5%)	14 (48.3%)
Prevalence reporting	31 (60.8%)	23 (79.3%)
Admission documentation	48 (94.1%)	28 (96.6%)
Discovery of pressure injury actions	50 (98%)	29 (100%)
Pressure injury location, small children	47 (92.2%)	29 (100%)
Pressure injury location, large children	31 (60.8%)	27 (93.1%)
Occurrence time frame	20 (39.2%)	24 (82.8%)
Braden Q scale high-risk score	26 (51%)	22 (75.9%)
Pediatric physiology	50 (98.1%)	29 (100%)
Braden Q scale risk assessment frequency	1 (2%)	11 (37.9%)
Nutrition	49 (96.1%)	26 (89.7%)
Interventions	47 (92.2%)	27 (93.1%)
Prevention strategies	50 (98.0%)	29 (100%)
Medical device assessments	48 (94.1%)	28 (96.6%)
Total knowledge assessment mean[a]	61.6%	79.5%

Note. Numbers and percentages reflect questions answered correctly by PICU nurses.
  [a] Total knowledge assessment mean reflects the average percentage of questions answered correctly by PICU nurses on the PICU pre and post pressure injury education assessments.

children ($t = 3.20$, $df = 28$; $P<.05$), pressure injury location on large children ($t = 4.82$, $df = 28$; $P<.05$), pediatric pressure injury occurrence time frame ($t = 5.44$, $df = 28$; $P<.05$), Braden Q scale high-risk score ($t = 3.03$, $df = 28$; $P<.05$), and Braden Q scale risk assessment frequency ($t = 5.49$, $df = 28$; $P<.05$). PICU nurses demonstrated a significant decrease in knowledge following the education session in regards to nutrition in PICU patients ($t = -2.38$, $df = 28$; $P<.05$). Overall, the education session significantly increased PICU nurses' knowledge on pediatric pressure injuries: t (28) = 9.19, $P<.001$, $d = 8.88$.

TURNING COMPLIANCE

PICU patient turning compliance before the delivery of pediatric pressure injury education to the PICU nursing team was 47% (**Table 4**). PICU patient turning compliance improved throughout the quality improvement project to 63%. This is a 34% increase in patient turning compliance from baseline. Turning compliance for PICU patients at high risk of developing pressure injuries increased from 36% to 67%.

NUTRITION CONSULTATION COMPLIANCE

The ordering of nutrition consultations for patients with a Braden Q scale risk score of 16 or less improved from 7% to 100% (**Table 5**). This significant increase from baseline is directly related to the implementation of the automatic ordering of nutrition

Table 3
PICU nursing staff knowledge assessment pre and post pressure injury education paired *t* test

	Preintervention (n = 29)	Postintervention (n = 29)	t	df	D[d]
Assessment Questions					
Causation	3 (10.3%)	16 (55.2%)	5.07[b]	28	1.12
Pediatric causation	7 (24.1%)	14 (48.3%)	3.37[b]	28	0.92
Risk factors	1 (3.4%)	16 (55.2%)	7.26[b]	28	2.0
Outcomes	8 (27.6%)	14 (48.3%)	2.38[b]	28	0.54
Prevalence reporting	17 (58.6%)	23 (79.3%)	2.19[b]	28	0.45
Admission documentation	28 (96.6%)	28 (96.6%)	0	28	—
Discovery of pressure injury actions	29 (100%)	29 (100%)	—	—	—
Pressure injury location, small children	24 (82.8%)	29 (100%)	3.20[b]	28	1.67
Pressure injury location, large children	16 (55.2%)	27 (93.1%)	4.82[b]	28	1.20
Occurrence time frame	10 (34.5%)	24 (82.8%)	5.44[b]	28	1.20
Braden Q scale high-risk score	14 (48.3%)	22 (75.9%)	3.03[b]	28	0.65
Pediatric physiology	29 (100%)	29 (100%)	—	—	—
Braden Q scale risk assessment frequency	0 (0%)	11 (37.9%)	5.49[b]	28	1.56
Nutrition	29 (100%)	26 (89.7%)	−2.38[b]	28	−1.08
Interventions	27 (93.1%)	27 (93.1%)	—	—	—
Prevention strategies	29 (100%)	29 (100%)	—	—	—
Medical device assessments	29 (100%)	28 (96.6%)	−1.32	28	−1.0
Total knowledge assessment mean[a]	60.85%	79.5%	9.19[c]	28	8.88

Note. Numbers and percentages reflect questions answered correctly by PICU nurses.
[a] Total knowledge assessment mean reflects the average percentage of questions answered correctly by PICU nurses on the PICU pre and post pressure injury education assessments.
[b] $P < .05$.
[c] $P < .001$.
[d] Cohen d effect size. Large effect is >0.8, medium effect is >0.5, and small effect is >0.2.

consultations in the electronic medical record on PICU patients with Braden Q scale scores 16 or less. Before the implementation of the electronic trigger, nurses had to request providers place an order for a nutrition consultation on a patient at high risk for developing pressure injuries.

Pressure Injury Weekly Incidence

The PICU pressure injury weekly incidence rate May 7, 2017, through May 13, 2017, before the delivery of pressure injury education to the PICU nursing staff was 8% (**Table 6**). The weekly PICU pressure injury incidence rate from June 4, 2017, through June 30, 2017, was 3%, which is a 63% decrease from baseline.

DISCUSSION

The PICU pressure injury incidence rate decreased from 8% to 3% during the quality improvement project, therefore the project aim was met. The decrease in the weekly

Table 4
PICU patient turning compliance

	Preintervention (n = 197)	Postintervention (n = 560)
Patients at low risk[a]	43 (43%)	148 (53%)
Patients at moderate risk[b]	45 (54%)	153 (64%)
Patients at high risk[c]	5 (36%)	49 (67%)
Total turning compliance[d]	93 (47%)	350 (63%)

Note. Preintervention time period was May 7, 2017, through May 13, 2017. Postintervention time period was June 5, 2017, through June 30, 2017.
[a] PICU patients with a Braden Q risk score of 23 or higher who were turned every 2 h during their stay.
[b] PICU patients with a Braden Q risk score between 17 and 22 who were turned every 2 h during their stay.
[c] PICU patients with a Braden Q risk score of 16 or less who were turned every 2 h during their stay.
[d] Percentage of PICU patients at mild, moderate, or high risk of developing pressure injuries who were turned every 2 h during their stay in the PICU.

pressure injury incidence rate should be interpreted with caution because the PICU pressure injury incidence rate has been dropping rapidly since January 2017. Several structure changes were implemented in January 2017 to better support pressure injury prevention efforts throughout the hospital and many of those changes have taken place on the PICU. The hospital and the PICU have experienced a 50% reduction in pressure injuries since the implementation of the structure changes. Hospital leaders should interpret the quality improvement findings as promising and continue to monitor pressure injury incidence rates.

The pressure injury education session results are significant; however, the sample size is not large enough to generalize the findings to the entire PICU staff. The knowledge assessment highlights several significant pediatric pressure injury knowledge gaps among PICU nurses. PICU nurses receive the same pressure injury education as the rest of the pediatric nurses at the hospital, therefore nursing leaders should consider assessing pediatric pressure injury knowledge throughout the hospital. Historically, pressure injury education at the pediatric hospital has been based on adult pressure injury prevention strategies and focused around properly staging pressure injuries on discovery. The knowledge assessment pretest findings imply PICU nurses know what to do to prevent pressure injuries, but they do not understand why. Pressure injury prevention interventions will remain tasks to PICU nurses until they

Table 5
Nutrition consultation ordering for PICU patients at high risk for pressure injuries

	Preintervention (n = 33)	Postintervention (n = 31)
Total nutrition consultation compliance	3 (9%)[a]	31 (100%)[a]

Note. Table shows the number and percentage of PICU patients with Braden Q scale risk scores of 16 or less with nutrition consultations ordered in their electronic medical records. Preintervention time period was from May 7, 2017, through May 13, 2017. Postintervention time period was June 20, 2017, through June 30, 2017.
[a] Percentage of PICU patients at high risk of developing pressure injuries who had a nutrition consultation ordered.

Table 6		
PICU pressure injury incidence		
	Preintervention[a] (n = 26)	Postintervention[b] (n = 100)
PICU pressure injury weekly incidence	2[c] (8%)	3[c] (3%)

[a] Preintervention time period was May 7, 2017, through May 13, 2017.
[b] Postintervention time period was June 4, 2017, through June 30, 2017.
[c] Number of pressure injuries stage 2, 3, 4, deep tissue injuries, and unstageable pressure injuries during the time frame.

understand the physiology and reasoning behind why the prevention strategies are appropriate and effective at reducing pediatric pressure injuries. Leaders must help nurses connect the why behind what they do.

Turning compliance improved during the quality improvement project. PICU nurses told the project leader they knew to turn patients routinely to prevent ventilator-associated pneumonia but confessed they had lost focus on turning patients to reduce pressure injuries. Repositioning patients to prevent ventilator-associated pneumonia often involves raising the head of the bed. This is counterproductive to preventing pressure injuries because of the increase in pressure on the sacrum with a higher head of bed. Nurses must use critical thinking in caring for their patients to assess their patient's risk for pressure injuries and ventilator-associated pneumonia in the PICU.

Historically, PICU providers and nursing staff have paid little attention to the important role nutrition plays in preventing pressure injuries. Therefore, it was not surprising that nutrition consultations were rarely ordered for patients at high risk for pressure injuries. PICU dieticians were eager to help but relied on providers to order nutrition consultations on patients at high risk for pressure injuries. PICU dieticians told the project leader they "never" talked about pressure injury risk or patient wound healing in medical team rounds before this quality improvement project because there was no trigger for them to consider it in their nutrition recommendations. Nutrition consultations are now routinely ordered and completed for all patients at high risk for pressure injuries in the PICU. The implementation of the automatic nutrition consultation order reduces the burden on the providers to place the order and allows the dieticians to function more effectively on the unit.

IMPACT OF RESULTS ON PRACTICE

The quality improvement project improved the quality of care being delivered to patients in the PICU by increasing nurses' knowledge of pediatric pressure injury risk factors and evidence-based prevention strategies, improving turning compliance, and implementing an electronic trigger to enhance nutrition support for patients at risk of developing pressure injuries. The quality improvement project also decreased preventable patient harm to PICU patients by decreasing the pressure injury incidence rate. The findings highlight the importance of ensuring staff nurses remain up to date on evidence-based practices for their patient populations. Pediatric pressure injury research is rapidly developing with a specific focus on effective medical device–related pressure injury prevention strategies. Nationally, it is common for adult pressure injury prevention strategies to be spread to pediatric facilities with the assumption pressure injuries in adults and pediatrics share the same causation, risk factors, and prevention strategies.[10,22] This one size fits all approach contributes to high pediatric pressure injury incidence rates in the PICU population because adult pressure injury prevention strategies are not aligned with pediatric pressure injury risk factors. This quality improvement project demonstrates PICU nurses are not knowledgeable on the growing body of evidence around pediatric pressure injury causation, risk factors, and prevention strategies. Thus, pediatric pressure injury research findings are not reaching their intended audiences. Health care leaders should focus resources on ensuring evidence is translated to practice and technology is leveraged to link risk assessment tools with evidence-based prevention strategies to guide clinical decision making and improve patient outcomes.

REFERENCES

1. Agency for Healthcare Research and Quality. Are we ready for this change? 2014. Available at: https://www.ahrq.gov/professionals/systems/hosptial/pressureulcertoolkit/putool1.html. Accessed September 20, 2016.
2. Institute of Healthcare Improvement. Relieve the pressure and reduce harm. 2016. Available at: http://www.ihi.org/resources/pages/improvementstories/relievethepressureandreduceharm.aspx. Accessed September 7, 2016.
3. National Pressure Ulcer Advisory Panel. NPUAP pressure injury stages. 2016. Available at: http://www.npuap.org/resources/educational-and-clinical-resources/npuap-pressure-injury-stages/. Accessed September 7, 2016.
4. Curley M, Quigley S, Lin M. Pressure ulcers in pediatric intensive care: incidence and associated factors. Pediatr Crit Care Med 2003;4:284–90.
5. Graves N, Birrell F, Whitby M. Effect of pressure ulcers on length of hospital stay. Infect Control Hosp Epidemiol 2005;26:293–7.
6. Institute of Medicine. To err is human: building a safer health system. 1999. Available at: http://www.nap.edu/books/0309068371/html. Accessed October 3, 2016.
7. Duncan K. Preventing pressure ulcers: the goal is zero. Jt Comm J Qual Patient Saf 2007;33:605–10.
8. The Joint Commission. 2016 National Patient Safety Goal Presentation. 2016. Available at: https://www.jointcommission.org/npsg_presentation/. Accessed September 20, 2016.
9. Noonan C, Quigley S, Curley M. Skin integrity in hospitalized infants and children: a prevalence survey. J Pediatr Nurs 2006;21:445–53.
10. Schindler C, Mikhailov T, Kuhn E, et al. Protecting fragile skin: nursing interventions to decrease development of pressure ulcers in pediatric intensive care. Am J Crit Care 2011;20:26–35.
11. Dixon M, Ratliff C. Pediatric pressure ulcer prevalence: one hospitals experience. Ostomy Wound Manage 2005;51:44–6.
12. Titler M, Kleiber C, Steelman V, et al. The Iowa model of evidence-based practice to promote quality care. Crit Care Nurs Clin North Am 2001;13:497–509.
13. Dang D, Melnyk B, Fineout-Overholt E, et al. Models to guide implementation and sustainability of evidence-based practice. In: Melnyk B, Fineout-Overholt E, editors. Evidence-based practice in nursing and healthcare. Philadelphia: Wolters Kluwer Health; 2015. p. 274–315.
14. Kiss E, Heiler M. Pediatric skin integrity practice guideline for institutional use: a quality improvement project. J Pediatr Nurs 2014;29:362–7.
15. Neiderhauser A, Lukas C, Parker V, et al. Comprehensive programs for preventing pressure ulcers: a review of the literature. Adv Skin Wound Care 2012;25:167–88.
16. Peterson J, Adlard K, Walti B, et al. Clinical nurse collaboration to recognize, prevent, and treat pediatric pressure ulcers. Clin Nurse Spec 2015;29:276–82.

17. Schindler C, Mikhailov T, Cashin S, et al. Under pressure: preventing pressure ulcers in critically ill infants. J Spec Pediatr Nurs 2013;18:329–41.

18. Visscher M, King A, Nie A, et al. A quality-improvement collaborative project to reduce pressure ulcers in PICUs. Pediatrics 2013;131:e1950–60.

19. Noonan C, Quigley S, Curley M. Using the Braden Q Scale to predict pressure ulcer risk in pediatric patients. J Pediatr Nurs 2011;26:566–75.

20. Institute for Healthcare Improvement. How to improve. 2017. Available at: http://www.ihi.org/resources/Pages/HowtoImprove/default.aspx. Accessed September 7, 2016.

21. Agency for Healthcare Research and Quality. How do we measure our pressure ulcer rates and practices?. 2014. Available at: https://www.ahrq.gov/professionals/systems/hospital/pressureulcertoolkit/putool5.html. Accessed September 12, 2016.

22. Reedy M, Gill S, Rochon P. Preventing pressure ulcers: a systematic review. JAMA 2006;296:974–84.

Screening for Social Determinants of Health at Well-Child Appointments
A Quality Improvement Project

Kimberly Higginbotham, DNP, APRN, CPNP, PMHS[a],*,
Terri Davis Crutcher, DNP, MSN, RN[b],
Sharon M. Karp, PhD, MSN, RN, CPNP-PC[c]

KEYWORDS

- Social determinants of health • Poverty • Children • Food insecurity
- Housing insecurity • Toxic stress • Quality improvement • Rural health clinic

KEY POINTS

- Poverty and related social determinants of health negatively impact the health and well-being of children.
- This quality improvement project identified approximately one in four children with unmet basic needs during well-child appointments.
- The short five-item FI and HI self-administered screening tool was easily implemented, maintaining the flow of well-child appointments in a primary care setting.

Children living in poverty are vulnerable to the adverse effects associated with unmet basic needs, such as food and housing.[1,2] Children depend on their families for basic needs.[3] Consequently, the inability of families to meet basic needs directly impacts the health and well-being of children.[4] Food insecurity (FI) and housing insecurity (HI) are two examples of social determinants of health (SDOH) that contribute to health disparities in childhood.[1] SDOH include five determinants (**Box 1**)[5]:

Poverty, a component of economic stability, is a strong determinant of health and associated with detrimental health outcomes during childhood extending into adulthood.[1,5–7] The Commission on Social Determinants of Health[8] suggests that disease leading to death occurs as the result of "the immediate and structural conditions in

Conflict of Interest: The author has no commercial or financial conflicts of interests to disclose. There is no funding for this quality improvement initiative.
[a] Cedarville University, School of Nursing, 251 N. Main Street, Cedarville, OH 45314, USA;
[b] Vanderbilt University School of Nursing, 222 Godchaux Hall, 461 21st Avenue South, Nashville, TN 37240, USA; [c] Vanderbilt University, School of Nursing, 461 21st Ave S., Nashville, TN 37240, USA
* Corresponding author.
E-mail address: higginjk@cedarville.edu

| Box 1 |
| Social determinants of health |

1. Economic stability

2. Education

3. Social and community context

4. Health and health care

5. Neighborhood and built environment

Data from Healthy People 2020. 2017. Available at: http://www.healthypeople.gov. Accessed February 2, 2017.

which people are born, grow, live, work, and age."[8] Childhood poverty alters early brain development through the mechanism of toxic stress.[9] Furthermore, there is increased evidence linking poverty in childhood with neuroendocrine dysregulation possibly leading to the development of chronic cardiovascular, immune, and psychiatric disorders.[1,10]

The American Academy of Pediatrics (AAP), Healthy People 2020, and the Robert Wood Johnson Foundation Commission to Build a Healthier America[1,5,11] recommend screening for SDOH in primary care. The AAP Policy on Health Equity emphasizes that primary care appointments are an opportunity to screen and address the social, economic, educational, and environmental needs of children and families.[6,12] Screening for unmet needs, such as food and housing, is an essential initiative in meeting the AAP policy guidelines that call for pediatric providers to intervene to reduce toxic stress.[1,6]

Evidence suggests that screening for social determinants should be comprehensive and should identify multiple needs, if they exist, simultaneously.[2,4,13] Screening is necessary before implementing interventions, such as connecting children and their families to resources.[3,4,6] Pediatric providers are positioned to identity unfavorable SDOH and resources available to alleviate the stress caused by unmet basic needs.[3,4,6] Despite the clear evidence pointing to the impact of social determinants on child health, few pediatric providers consistently address SDOH during routine primary care visits.[6]

BACKGROUND

The US Census Bureau uses dollar value thresholds to determine poverty estimates.[14] The poverty thresholds vary according to the size and composition of a family.[14] The US Census Bureau 2017 data indicate nearly 39% of US children lived in households in or around poverty levels.[14] Of those 28 million US children younger than 18, upward of 8% lived in households in deep poverty (income less than 50% of their poverty threshold level), and 17.5% lived in households below poverty (income less than 100% of their poverty threshold level).[14] It is estimated that 37% of all children live in poverty for some period during their childhood.[15] Poverty is an adverse SDOH restricting the ability of families to meet basic needs, such food and housing, which negatively impacts physical, emotional, cognitive, and behavioral outcomes of children.[1,6,7]

The US Department of Agriculture (USDA) defines FI as the "lack of access to enough food to fully meet basic nutritional needs because of insufficient resources."[16] Household FI includes low food security and very low food security.[16] Low food security includes reduction in quality, variety, and desirability of food without reduction in quantity; very low food security includes altered patterns of eating accompanied by a decrease in food intake in addition to reduction in quality, variety, and desirability.[16] The demographic of FI reaches outside of urban settings into the suburbs and rural areas, which were once considered unaffected by this growing problem.[17] In 2015, the USDA reported 15.8 million US households met the USDA definition of an FI household.[18] The AAP Council on Community Pediatrics and Committee on Nutrition[1,17] suggest a correlation of multiple adverse health outcomes with FI at all levels. Children living in FI households are susceptible to the harmful effects of poor nutrition, which can lead to negative psychological, behavioral, and cognitive outcomes.[19]

The US Department of Housing and Urban Development definition of HI encompasses steep housing cost in proportion to income, substandard housing quality, unstable neighborhoods, overcrowding, or homelessness.[20] Cutts and colleagues[21] linked HI with measures of poor health, and growth and development alterations in young children. They further suggest there was a stronger relation with fair/poor child health associated with multiple moves rather than overcrowding.[21] In addition, they identified HI as a salient indicator for FI.[21]

To assess and address the unmet basic needs of young children receiving care in a rural health clinic (RHC) a quality improvement (QI) project was implemented. Comprehensive primary care and preventative health care services, such as well-child care, episodic care, and behavioral health care, are provided at this RHC. This QI project focused on the implementation of FI and HI screening and referral process during well-child appointments.

METHODOLOGY

The Model for Improvement[22] provided a methodology for the implementation of this QI project. The Model for Improvement has two components including fundamental questions and the Plan-Do-Study-Act (PDSA) cycle. The Model for Improvement addresses three fundamental questions: (1) what are we trying to accomplish, (2) how will we know that a change is an improvement, and (3) what change can we make that will result in improvement.[22]

To address the first question (what are we trying to accomplish)[22] this QI project aimed to initiate FI and HI screening to 100% of children between the ages of 1 week and 5 years of age during well-child appointments. Subsequently, to answer the second question (how will we know that a change is an improvement)[22] the QI project measured the number of children ages 1 week to 5 years of age seen for well-child appointments and screened for FI and HI; and the number of referrals made for families who screened positive for FI and/or HI. No intentional screening for FI and HI existed at the RHC, so this QI project used the PDSA cycle to make an initial change on a small scale. To answer the third question (what change can we make that will result in improvement)[22] this QI project initiated the following changes: developed an evidenced-based FI and HI screening tool; defined the process for FI and HI screening related to clinic flow; and developed a one-page community resource guide and a protocol for follow-up of families identified as food and housing insecure.

At the time of the project, there were five pediatric providers including two pediatricians, one nurse practitioner, one licensed independent social worker, and one child psychologist providing mental health and behavioral counseling services. The composition of the project team allowed for clerical and clinical representation, which included a receptionist, registered nurse (RN), medical assistant (MA), two pediatricians, and pediatric nurse practitioner (project leader). The following outlines the PDSA cycle for this QI project.

A key step in the initial planning phase included the identification of evidence-based FI and HI screening tools and acquiring permission for screening tool use. Effective identification of FI included use of a reliable and valid two-item screen. Hager, and colleagues[23] developed a two-item FI tool from the USDA 18-item Household Food Security Survey, which is considered the gold standard in assessment of household food security. Affirmative response to either of these questions "Within the past 12 months, were you ever worried whether your food would run out before you got money to buy more" and "Within the past 12 months, did the food you bought not last and you did not have money to get more?"[23] indicates positive FI. The two-question FI screen is a valid tool with 97% sensitivity and 83% specificity.[23] The AAP Council on Community Pediatrics, Committee on Nutrition Policy Statement[17] practice level recommendations include incorporating the two-question validated screening tool at scheduled health maintenance appointments and identifying community resources for positive FI screen.

Using the US Department of Housing and Urban Development HI definition, Cutts and colleagues[21] published a cross-sectional study using a three-item HI screen that includes questions regarding crowding ("within the past 12 months there were two or more people per bedroom?"), doubling up ("within the past 12 months we were temporarily staying with another family or had another family staying with us?"), and frequent moving ("within the past 12 months we moved more than once?"). Bailey and colleagues[24] published a study referencing the HI psychometric from Cutts and colleagues[21] of overcrowding and multiple moves. For the purpose of this QI project, HI did not focus on the quality or cost of housing and instead used Cutts and colleagues's[21] published indicator of HI as overcrowding, including doubling up, and multiple moves. The project leader obtained permission from Dr Diana Cutts for use of the three-item HI screening tool for the purpose of this QI project.

Further considerations in the planning phase involved obtaining university institutional review board approval, gaining stakeholder support, identifying community agencies, and developing a one-page food and housing community resource guide. The project team determined a process for integrating the screening tool and community resource guide into the flow of the well-child appointment. Before project implementation, the project team was provided with details of the purpose of the tool, how to score the tool, and of the standardized screening process.

The Do phase began with implementing FI and HI screening and providing a community resource guide to families during a 3-week period of time. The RN and MA assisted with the patient flow by giving the HI and FI screening tool to the parents/guardians during the check-in process, retrieving and reviewing the screening tool, alerting the providers of positive screening, and providing the community resource guide to families that screened positive for FI and/or HI. The five-item, self-administered FI and HI tool included a statement ("in order to make sure you are aware of the community resources available to you, please answer the following questions") that the staff used to introduce the screening tool to families. White, English speaking, and low socioeconomic status families comprised most of the patient population. Exclusion criteria included an adult present for the well-child appointment not living in the household with the child.

The Study phase involved completion of data analysis. During this phase, the project leader summarized the data and determined if the aim of the project was achieved. The data analysis for this project contributed to an increased awareness of the unmet needs of the RHC patient population.

During the Act phase of the PDSA cycle, the project team reviewed the data analysis and determined that the FI and HI screening process assisted in the identification of families at risk for unmet basic needs. Following the data collection, the project team discussed ways to integrate FI and HI screening during well-child appointments as part of the standard of care during health maintenance appointments. Also, the project team discussed extending the screening to families with children seen for well-child and new appointments. As part of the Act phase, the project team reviewed the screening rates to determine ways to improve FI and HI screening. In addition, the project team discussed a process to determine if families used suggested referrals.

RESULTS

Descriptive statistics provided demographic data specific to the patient population at the RHC. During the project implementation period, 93 out of a total of 133 well-child appointments were scheduled for children from birth through age 5 years. There were 84 opportunities to screen for FI and HI, because nine patients did not keep their appointment. In total, 63% (n = 53) of patients/families were screened for FI and HI, because 31 patients and families did not receive the screening tool. All 53 patients/ families agreed to answer the five question FI and HI screening tool. There were 5% (n = 3) newborns, 54% (n = 29) infants, 32% (n = 17) toddlers, and 7.5% (n = 4) pre-schoolers represented in the 53 well-child appointments.

Almost 17% (16.9%; n = 9) screened positive for FI, reflecting FI in 33% (n = 1) of the newborns, 17.2% (n = 5) of the infants, 17.6% (n = 3) of the toddlers, and 0% (n = 0) of the preschoolers. The rate of FI total at the RHC is greater than the US (13.7%) and Ohio (16.1%) levels.[16,25] Nearly 19% (18.8%; n = 10) screened positive for HI, identified in 0% (n = 0) of the newborns, 17.2% (n = 5) of the infants, 23.5% (n = 4) of the toddlers, and 25% (n = 1) of the preschoolers. The HI total at the RHC is greater than the Ohio (15%) housing problem level.[25] Results found 11.3% (n = 6) positive for both FI and HI, represented in 0% (n = 0) of the newborns, 10.3% (n = 3) of the infants, 17.6% (n = 3) of the toddlers, and 0% (n = 0) of the preschoolers.

Staff screening rate for administering the screening tool was 63% overall, because there were 31 missed opportunities (37%) for FI and HI screening. The screening rate was 68% in Week 1, 45% in Week 2, and 77.4% in Week 3. The project leader re-evaluated the PDSA cycle when the screening rate dropped during Week 2, and met with staff to discuss missed opportunities for screening and ways to improve the process. The staff reported that human error, forgetting, was the main reason screening tools were not given to patients. To increase the screening rate, the project leader placed blank FI/HI screening tools in a brightly colored folder by the RN and MA workstation. The project leader reminded everyone of the goal of screening 100% of the patients and distributing the resource guide to families that screened positive. The screening rate in Week 3 improved to 77%. Of the 13 families screening positive for FI and/or HI, 85% were given a resource guide. One family was not given a community resource guide and one family left without the guide they had received.

DISCUSSION AND PRACTICE IMPLICATIONS

This QI initiative positively enhanced well-child care for children from newborn through 5 years of age at this RHC in several ways. Before the initiation of this QI project, there was no formal process for identifying and referring children and families with unmet basic needs. The intentional screening for SDOH (FI and HI) in this RHC went from roughly 0% to overall 63% within the timeframe of this project.

The screening yielded a high percentage of children and families (24.5%; n = 13) at the RHC with unmet basic needs. The data from the QI project at this RHC are compelling because of the strong scientific evidence regarding the detrimental effects of FI and HI. FI is a marker for household dysfunction and a risk factor for childhood toxic stress, altered brain development, and poor outcomes into adulthood.[26] Furthermore, the negative effects of stress associated with HI are a precursor to chronic disease in adulthood.[21] This project identified 11.3% (n = 6) of families who screened positive for both FI and HI (n = 3 infants and n = 3 toddlers). The presence of both FI and HI place very young children at increased risk for poor health and development.[1,17,21] In addition, it has been established that early childhood deprivation predicts morbidity in adulthood.[27] When families encounter cumulative hardship, they must make difficult decisions whether to pay rent or buy food.[28] Consequently, the inability to consistently provide basic needs creates stress in families and contributes to toxic stress.[1]

This QI project facilitated the identification of children in need of receiving additional support from resources, such as food banks, social services, and federally funded programs. This project provided families a community resource guide as a mechanism to promote the receipt of necessary resources to meet basic needs. Studies demonstrate that screening and referring those in need to community programs or agencies results in acquisition of resources.[4,13,19]

Nurse practitioners are positioned to lead QI initiatives directed toward improving patient outcomes. This QI initiative, led by a nurse practitioner, demonstrated the feasibility of incorporating a simplified screening and community resource referral process into the well-child appointments at an RHC. A self-administered screening tool provided a nonthreatening mechanism to gather information that assisted the provider in determining patient and family basic needs. Of the 53 patients/families given the FI and HI screening tool, 100% agreed to participate.

Strengths and Limitations of Quality Improvement Project

One of the most significant strengths of this project was that it aligned with the AAP, Healthy People 2020, and Robert Wood Johnson Foundation Commission to Build a Healthier America recommendation to screen for SDOH in the primary care setting.[1,5,13] The use of a short five-item self-administered FI and HI screening tool demonstrated the feasibility of maintaining and sustaining the flow of well-child appointments. In addition, the QI initiative secured an intentional mechanism to provide a community resource guide to facilitate the receipt of unmet basic needs. The synthesis of literature for this project yielded a gap in the knowledge of the FI and HI needs of rural families. The results of this project confirmed the consistent prevalence of FI and HI in the pediatric population in the rural pediatric primary care setting.

There were several limitations of this QI project. One was the number of missed screening opportunities (38%) because of human error. Another limitation of this project was the follow-up regarding the acquisition of resources to meet basic needs. Because of the limited length of time for this QI project, it was not feasible for the project team to follow up with families regarding resources or to determine if obtaining resources helped to address unmet basic needs.

SUMMARY

The strong recommendations to screen for unmet needs related to SDOH and the evidence demonstrating adverse health outcomes of poverty provide a persuasive reason to screen and refer those in need. Because child health has been identified as a predictor of adult health,[29] pediatric providers have a pivotal role in health care. Therefore, interventions directed toward early childhood are critical and must be guided by evidence; motivated by moral, ethical, and professional obligation; and focused toward improving population outcomes.

REFERENCES

1. Council on Community Pediatrics. Poverty and child health in the United States. Pediatrics 2016;137:1–14.
2. Garg R, Toy S, Yorghos T, et al. Addressing social determinants of health at well child care visits: a cluster RCT. Pediatrics 2015;135:2.
3. Fazalullasha F, Taras J, Morinis J, et al. From office tools to community supports: the need for infrastructure to address the social determinants of health in paediatric practice. Paediatr Child Health 2014;19:195–9.
4. Garg A, Butz AM, Dworkin PH, et al. Screening for basic social needs at a medical home for low-income children. Clin Pediatr 2009;48(1):32–6.
5. Healthy people 2020. 2017. Available at: http://www.healthypeople.gov. Accessed February 2, 2017.
6. Chung EK, Siegel BS, Garg A, et al. Screening for social determinants of health among children and families living in poverty: a guide for clinicians. Curr Probl Pediatr Adolesc Health Care 2016;46:135–53.
7. Brooks-Gunn J, Duncan GJ. The effects of poverty on children. Future Child 1997;7:55–71.
8. Marmot M, Friel S, Bell R, et al. Closing the gap in a generation: health equity through action on the social determinants of health. Lancet 2008;372:1661–9.
9. Pascoe JM, Wood DL, Duffee JH, et al. Mediators and adverse effects of child poverty in the United States. Pediatrics 2016;137:1–11.
10. Garner AS, Shonkoff JP, Siegel BS, et al. Early childhood adversity, toxic stress, and the role of the pediatrician: translating developmental science into lifelong health. Pediatrics 2012;129:224–30.
11. Robert Wood Johnson Foundation, 2014. Robert Wood Johnson Foundation Commission to build a healthier America. Available at: http://www.rwjf.org/en/library/collections/commission.html. Accessed January 20, 2017.
12. Cheng T, Emmanuel MA, Levy DJ, et al. Child health disparities: what can a clinician do? Pediatrics 2015;136:961–8.
13. Hassan A, Scherer EA, Pikcilingis A, et al. Improving social determinants of health, effectiveness of a web-based intervention. Am J Prev Med 2015;49(6):822–31.
14. United States Census Bureau. 2018. Available at: https://www.census.gov/data/tables/2018/demo/income-poverty/p60-263.html. Accessed October 21, 2018.
15. Ratcliffe C, McKernan SM. Childhood poverty persistence: facts and consequences. Urban Institute Brief. 2010. Available at: http://www.urban.org/UploadedPDF/412126-poverty-persistence.pdf. Accessed January 20, 2017.
16. United States Department of Agriculture, 2015. Available at: http://www.ers.usda.gov/topics/food-nutrition-assistance/food-security-in-the-us/definitions-of-food-security.aspx. Accessed January 20, 2017.
17. Council on Community Pediatrics and Committee on Nutrition. Promoting food security for all children. Pediatrics 2015;136:e1431–8.
18. Coleman-Jensen A, Gregory C, Singh A. Household food security in the United States in 2013. Washington, DC: US Department of Agriculture, Economic Research Service; 2014. Publication no. ERR-173.

19. Burkhardt MC, Beck AF, Conway PH, et al. Enhancing accurate identification of food insecurity using quality-improvement techniques. Pediatrics 2012;129: e504–10.

20. Johnson A, Meckstroth A. Ancillary services to support welfare to work. Washington, DC: U.S. Department of Health and Human Services; 1998. Available at: http://aspe,hhs.gov/hsp/isp/ancillary.

21. Cutts DB, Meyers AF, Black MM, et al. US Housing insecurity and the health of very young children. Am J Public Health 2011;101(8):1508–14.

22. Institute for Healthcare Improvement: associates in process improvement. 2017. Available at: http://www.apiweb.org. Accessed February 2, 2017.

23. Hager ER, Quigg AM, Black MM, et al. Development and validity of a 2-item screen to identify families at risk for food insecurity. Pediatrics 2010;126:e26–32.

24. Bailey KR, Cook JT, Ettinger de Cuba S, et al. Development of an index of subsidized housing availability and its relationship to housing insecurity. Housing Policy Debate 2015;26:172–87.

25. Country Health Rankings. 2017. Available at: http://www.countyhealthrankings. org. Accessed January 20, 2017.

26. Garner AS. Applying an ecobiodevelopmental framework to food insecurity: more than simply food for thought. J Appl Res Child 2012;3:1–5.

27. Evans G, Kim P. Childhood poverty, chronic stress, self-regulation, and coping. Child Dev Perspect 2013;7:43–8.

28. Knowles M, Rabinowich J, Ettinger de Cuba S, et al. "Do you wanna breathe or eat?": parent perspectives on child health consequences of food insecurity, trade-offs, and toxic stress. Matern Child Health J 2015;20:25–32.

29. American Academy of Pediatrics. Blueprint for children how the next president can build a foundation for a healthy future. 2016. Available at: http://www.aap. org/en-us/transitions/Pages/blueprint-for-children.aspx. Accessed January 20, 2017.

Diabetes Self-management Education Provision by an Interprofessional Collaborative Practice Team

A Quality Improvement Project

Adelaide N. Harris, DNP, MSN, MEd, RN

KEYWORDS

- Diabetes • Diabetes self-management education • Self-care behavior
- Interprofessional collaborative practice

KEY POINTS

- Diabetes is a prevalent disease.
- Diabetes requires people to gain knowledge to manage their condition.
- The shift in diabetes care is to focus teaching on self-management.

INTRODUCTION

Diabetes is a major health problem and an increasingly prevalent disease in the United States, affecting 9.3% of the adult population.[1,2] Insulin is a hormone produced by the pancreas and acts like a key to let blood sugar into the cells in the body for use as energy.[2] People with diabetes either do not make enough insulin (type 1 diabetes mellitus) or cannot use insulin properly (type 2 diabetes mellitus [T2DM]).[2] If you have T2DM, cells do not normally respond to insulin; this is called insulin resistance.[3] T2DM accounts for 90% to 95% of all diagnoses of diabetes.[1] The risk of developing diabetes is increased among Hispanics and blacks.[2]

It is important that patients with diabetes understand how to manage their care effectively. Knowledge of diabetes self-management is needed not only for providers and payers but also most importantly for patients, who have an essential role in managing their disease. There is strong evidence that diabetes self-management education (DSME) programs have beneficial effects on physical and emotional outcomes, along with improved health-related quality of life.[3] The increase in the individual and

The author has nothing to disclose.
Clinical Nursing, College of Nursing, University of Cincinnati, Academic Health Center, 3110 Vine Street, PO Box 210038, Cincinnati, OH 45221, USA
E-mail address: Adelaide.Harris@uc.edu

public health burden of diabetes makes it important to assess, prevent, and treat complications that may occur related to diabetes in the future.[4] The role of nurses in health promotion is essential to educate and engage patients in self-care.[4]

DESCRIPTION OF PROBLEM

Evidence shows DSME by health care providers improves disease management and quality of life and reduces hospitalizations.[3] Patients diagnosed with diabetes may lack proper knowledge to manage their disease effectively. Lack of knowledge may also pose a risk for developing complications of diabetes. DSME is a crucial element of care for patients with diabetes to delay or prevent complications of the disease.[5]

DSME is a process through which people with diabetes are educated about behavior and lifestyle modifications to manage their disease[6,7] and supported by evidenced-based standards to assist nurses in teaching patients.[6,7] Self-management support as evidenced by DSME engages patients with chronic disease, such as diabetes, in decision making that improves health-related behaviors and clinical outcomes on an ongoing basis.[5]

In today's complex health environment, interprofessional collaboration is one of the hallmarks of successful health care innovations.[8,9] The Institute of Medicine report, *The Future of Nursing*, calls for nurses to take a leadership role in the changing health care system.[8,9] Interprofessional collaboration refers to the interactions between individuals who bring their expertise from various educational backgrounds, experience, and values to the processes of delivering care.[6] It is important for health professionals to engage in collaborative interprofessional practice to achieve optimal health outcomes. The interprofessional collaborative practice (IPCP) team members identified for this project consisted of a family nurse practitioner, a registered nurse, a pharmacist, and a social worker.

PURPOSE OF PROJECT

The purpose of this quality improvement (QI) project was to increase the provider adherence rate of documenting patient-DSME (P-DSME) with T2DM patients at a health center.

AIM AND OBJECTIVES

The aim of the QI project was to implement a documentation education program for the IPCP to increase the provider adherence rate of P-DSME documentation on the diabetes flow sheet from 0% to 100% for patients whose hemoglobin A_{1C} (HbA$_{1C}$) levels are 8% or greater at the health center over a 60-day period. The patient education provided by the IPCP to patients with diabetes is noted as P-DSME. The provision of DSME is accomplished through 1-hour education sessions.

The objectives were to educate the IPCP on support informed decision making, self-care behaviors, problem solving, and collaboration with the IPCP; improve health outcomes and quality of life; and improve the IPCP' assessment and evaluation of patients' achievement of the American Association of Diabetes Educator 7 (AADE7) diabetes self-care behaviors. The providers' documentation on patients' DSME served as measurement of achievement of the AADE7 self-care behaviors.

SOCIAL DETERMINANTS OF HEALTH FRAMEWORK

The social determinants of health framework provide an understanding of the living conditions and other social, economic, and cultural factors that influence the health of patients. Social determinants affect how one lives and have an impact on health out-comes.[10] Social determinants of health play an important role in the targeted popula-tion, where a majority of residents are living below the poverty level line and meet the criteria for classification as a vulnerable population. Among the social determinants of a vulnerable population are being part of a minority population, poverty-level income, lack of education, lack of accessibility to healthy foods, and living with more than 1 illness. Each of these social determinants negatively affects health outcomes, and, in combination, vulnerability increases.[11,12] Knowledge of social determinants of health informs holistic caring for patients with a chronic disease like diabetes.[11]

The health center IPCP must take into consideration the social, cultural, economic, and physical factors affecting their patients' health. Re-educating the IPCP includes increasing awareness of health determinants in assessing and planning an effective intervention for patients. The team must be knowledgeable of multiple factors, including environmental factors, such as resources availability, quality of schools, safe and livable housing environmental factors, clean air, clean water, healthy foods, and access to health care. These conditions affect self-care/management, quality of life, and risk of poor health outcomes in patients with diabetes in this project.

NEEDS ASSESSMENT

The director of nursing identified the patients with elevated HbA_{1C} that was poorly controlled (ie, HbA_{1C} >8%). The evidence within the agency revealed that improved diabetes education could reduce the risk of developing diabetes related complica-tions. Prior to initiation of this QI project, 10 chart audits revealed no documentation of DSME and lack of performance in the National Committee for Quality Assurance guidelines specific for best practice in diabetes care management, especially for documentation of diabetes education. This project lead deemed it necessary in the in-terest of the patients to improve documentation by educating the IPCP on the AADE7 self-care behaviors in the provision and documentation of diabetes education to high-risk patients with diabetes. As a result, a QI project was developed and implemented to improve documentation of the DSME. This QI project targeted the IPCP team mem-ber's provision of DSME interventions and documentation.

METHODS
Project Design

The design for this project was QI using the model for improvement (MFI) to direct the project work. The MFI is composed of 2 parts of equal importance: (1) the 3 funda-mental questions and (2) the plan-do-study-act (PDSA) cycle of improvement.[13]

The 3 fundamental questions are What change are we trying to accomplish? How will we know that a change is an improvement? and What change can we make that will result in improvement? The MFI has been used to accelerate process improvement by numerous health care organizations successfully.[13,14] The second part of the MFI, the PDSA cycle, consists of small tests of change in a real-world setting.[13]

Plan

Evidence supports that targeted DSME improves patient outcomes, including reduc-tion and lowering of frequent hospitalizations and diabetes complications.[3,15] The aim for this QI project was to increase the provider adherence rate of P-DSME documen-tation in patients with T2DM whose HbA_{1C} levels are 8% or greater. The project's change was to educate the members of the health center's IPCP on DSME and the importance of providing and documenting P-DSME. The project lead established a list of patients with HbA_{1C} 8% and higher in the past 6 months at the health center. In addition, the project lead established a baseline of documentation of P-DSME on the flow sheet of patients with HbA_{1C} 8% and higher from the list of patients at the clinic.

Do

The IPCP participated in the IPCP-DSME session conducted by the project lead to review DSME and the importance of its provision and documentation. The education session provided current evidence-based practice recommendations for patients with T2DM (Appendix 1). The education session also provided current evidence-based knowledge on diabetes self-management. The AADE7 topics and the DSME flow sheet currently used for documentation of DSME were reviewed. The AADE7 consist of low-literacy, 1-page tear-off sheets on each of 7 topics. The AADE7 topics reviewed in the IPCP-DSME session included healthy eating, being active, monitoring blood sugars, taking medications, problem solving, healthy coping, and reducing risks (Appendix 2). The IPCP-DSME education intervention lasted approximately 30 minutes, after which the IPCP had the opportunity to ask questions.

Study

The diabetes quality measure was defined by the rate of P-DSME documentation by the IPCP for patients aged 22 years through 81 years with T2DM with HbA_{1C} 8% or higher. The operational definition of the outcome measure was used to define data points on the run chart. The same operational definition was used to define data points on run charts throughout the project. The operational definition is described as follows:

1. Denominator: patients with T2DM, 22 years to 81 years old, with HbA_{1C} 8% or higher seen in the health center over the past week; numerator: the number of "yes" response documented on the diabetes flow sheet in the electronic health record (EHR) clinic chart
2. Measure: rate of clinic charts with completed DSME
3. Population targeted: patients 22 years to 81 years of age with a diagnosis of T2DM and a HbA_{1C} level 8% or greater
4. To obtain baseline data: the first 12 data points before the intervention established a baseline median[16,17]
5. Goal: 100% increase in P-DSME documentation
6. Project aims: to increase the frequency of the provision of DSME to individuals with diabetes and its documentation by the IPCP in the EHR flow sheet at the health center

Postintervention data were obtained during chart reviews to ascertain compliance with documentation of P-DSME. When subsequent chart reviews after the IPCP-DSME session revealed continued deficiencies in documentation, the project lead provided additional 1-on-1 education to IPCP on the importance of P-DSME provision and the use of the AADE7 DSME self-care behaviors to assist them in providing patients with information on the topics essential to diabetes self-management.

Study

Baseline data were obtained before the initiation of the project. The number of data points collected was displayed on a run chart (approach chosen for assessing impact of intervention). The run chart displayed a baseline on IPCP documentation of P-DSME on the diabetes flow sheet (**Fig. 1**). The X axis of the run chart represents clinic days as the date of the visit and the Y axis represents the rate of documented DSME per 10 charts. Retrospective chart review was conducted for 10 clinic days

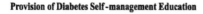

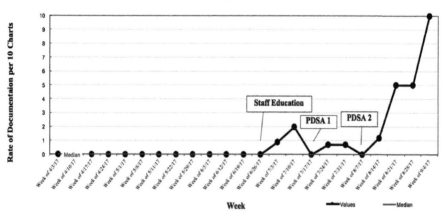

Fig. 1. Run chart of IPCP documentation.

before the intervention for patients with T2DM and HbA$_{1C}$ 8% or greater at the health center. The provision of DSME was accomplished through the collaboration with patients and the IPCP; for example, the family nurse practitioner, registered nurses, pharmacists, and social worker. The retrospective chart review verified the prediction was correct; there was no documentation of the provision of P-DSME in the EHR. The baseline median line was displayed on the run chart, representing the aggregate for all IPCP.

The post-education intervention data collected were obtained through EHR chart review of patients seen by IPCP team member each week to ascertain the provision and documentation of P-DSME. To conduct the chart reviews, the project manager received a list of patients who had diabetes clinic visits the prior week and who met the project criteria from the clinic nurse administrator. The patient synopsis data received included the EHR number of the patients (converted to patient code number for record keeping) and date of the recent clinic visit. The project manager reviewed the current visit to verify if there was documentation of DSME for the previous visit and which DSME topic is present.

The first test of change using the PDSA cycle was conducted post–education session with the IPCP. The first PDSA cycle determined there was a change in providers' behavior in providing and documenting P-DSME. The group education session showed positive results, and, when the measure began to move to accomplish the aim, the first cycle was completed. The improvement was not sustained, however, and a new PDSA cycle was initiated. In the second PDSA cycle, the project manager provided 1-on-1 reinforcement of documentation that was present and additional education when it was not to individual care providers. The second PDSA cycle with on 1-on-1 reinforcement or additional education reminders moved the measure toward the intended outcome measure. After the desired outcome measure was achieved, there was no need to test and evaluate a different approach in a new cycle. The run chart indicated when and what tests of change were initiated. The annotation on the run chart of P-DSME documentation displays each week's result and the date that each test of change intervention was implemented and its outcome, for example, the rate of patients with completed documentation.

The project lead asked IPCP during each PDSA cycle about barriers to providing P-DSME. The barriers expressed by the IPCP were documented and content analyzed using a qualitative conventional approach. In the conventional content analysis, the categorical codes come directly from the qualitative data that had been collected from the participants.[18] As discussed previously, in this project, these data were the IPCP' expressed barriers to the provision and documentation of DSME. Themes in their barriers to care were identified and reported were lack of training about DSME documentation on the diabetes flow sheet, lack of documentation of DSME plans and goals in collaboration with patients, lack of time to document P-DSME, lack of educational materials on site, and resources for self-management support.

Act

The leadership team was informed of problematic issues affecting DSME documentation. This then led the director of nursing to place a greater emphasis on adherence to completion of documentation on the DSME flow sheet by IPCP.

Although the AADE7 topics areas, listed previously, provide an outline for the education session, it is important that the content is tailored to meet patient needs and be adapted as necessary for age, cultural factors, health literacy, and comorbidities.[5] Although there are commonalities, each patient situation has distinct characteristics that require the IPCP to approach each patient without making assumptions as to the patient's and family's background, resources, and capability to learn to improve health outcomes. There is evidence that P-DSME can increase knowledge, modify self-care behaviors, and improve outcomes, such as lowering HbA_{1C} and reducing the related complications of diabetes.[19] The IPCP may lack knowledge and understanding about the ethnic population to sufficiently engage patients.[19] The IPCP-DSME included information about cultural and health beliefs that have an impact on care and P-DSME interventions that address dietary practices in an ethnic population.

A critical element in the teaching process is mutually establishing goals, so that patient, family, and staff are working together to achieve a common goal (short term or long term). Another aspect of the education process is to engage patients to identify their concerns, questions, and priority needs, to help them attain their health-related goals. The importance of patient factors, such as age, race, culture, health beliefs, and those described in the Maslow hierarchy of needs, are additional topics to be incorporated in the education of the IPCP.[3,20,21]

RESULTS

The results from this QI project showed in an increased rate of 100% (10 per 10 charts) in the IPCP' documentation of DSME on the diabetes flow sheet. The frequency data from the diabetes flow sheet documentation were presented in a run chart that displayed trends in improvements in the documentation that may have occurred in the provision of P-DSME by the IPCP after the IPCP-DSME intervention.

The run chart used for this project graphically displayed data plotted over time and yielded data to make conclusions and detect process improvement. To establish a baseline, at least 12 or more data points add a horizontal line representing the median that shows half the data points are above and half are below.[16,17] The same operational definition was used to define data points on run charts throughout the project. The target population was patients 18 years to 81 years of age with a diagnosis of T2DM and an HbA_{1C} level 8% or greater.

The baseline/preintervention diabetes self-management documentation rate for patients with T2DM was zero, indicating no provision of P-DSME on the flow sheet. The project lead did outcome measures were obtained through weekly chart reviews postintervention. Weekly chart reviews were performed for 10 weeks postintervention and showed positive trends. Two weeks out of 10 weeks there was no P-DSME documentation, and PDSA cycles were conducted. There were some unforeseen circumstances and staff performance issues that led to no documentation, zero rates. The run chart showed improved documentation post–PDSA cycle, return to no documentation, and improved documentation post–PDSA cycle 2 chart review (see **Fig. 1**). The Y axis displayed rate of documentation per charts. The rate was 5 charts per 10 charts per 1 week of a month of the project; patients with T2DM charts had DSME documentation on the flow sheet. The next month retrospective chart review revealed an increased rate to 10 charts in the P-DSME documentation of the flow sheet by the IPCP (see **Fig. 1**).

LIMITATIONS

The QI pilot project had a few limitations. The convenience sample of IPCP at the neighborhood health center was the target population for diabetes education by the project lead. A larger sample that was more representative of interprofessional health care providers from more than 1 Cincinnati health care center would have benefited as a population health approach to diabetes care measures, such as educational documentation. Short change period project occurred in only 1 setting, so the results are not generalizable.

Other limitations were the IPCP did not consistently document DSME at the point of care on the DSME flowsheet at the neighborhood health center, even though they found it time-saving. Access to the current diabetes flow sheet on the patient chart took some time if it was not previously uploaded in the chart at the point of care in real time. Therefore, documentation was done in other areas of the chart.

IPCP documentation of DSME on the diabetes flow sheet can be improved with targeted educational efforts, but the support of the agency leadership is imperative to sustain adherence. By increasing the engagement of IPCP in the self-care AADE7 documentation, patient outcomes are further improved, thereby decreasing the likelihood of complications from diabetes.

IMPLICATIONS FOR PRACTICE

The clinic operates under the patient-centered medical home Model which ensures care high-quality, cost effective and individualized care.[22] The health center is a federally qualified health center and is a patient-centered clinic. Through a patient-centered approach, an interprofessional team provides comprehensive care across the continuum of life and manages chronic diseases, such as diabetes, by providing patients with preventive health education.[23]

A nurse's role in the promotion of health involves proper knowledge of diseases and their treatment but also awareness of the social determinants influencing health to care for patients holistically. The nurse can also use evidence-based practice standards to prevent diabetes-related complications. Improving relationships and effective communication between health care providers and patients can have a positive impact on health outcomes and improve patient and staff satisfaction.

SUMMARY

The aim of this QI project was to implement a documentation education process for the IPCP to increase the rate of provider adherence with P-DSME documentation on the diabetes flow sheet form from 0% to 100% for patients with T2DM whose HbA$_{1C}$ levels were 8% or greater at the health center over a 60-day period. This project's aim is significant because diabetes is a major health concern and has an increasing prevalence in the United States and the city neighborhood of Cincinnati, Ohio.[2,24,25]

An interprofessional approach among health care providers has been reported to improve patients' disease management and quality of life and reduce hospitalizations.[3] Patients diagnosed with diabetes may lack proper knowledge to manage their disease effectively. This lack of knowledge also may increase the risk of developing complications of diabetes. DSME is a crucial element of care for patients with diabetes to delay or prevent complications of the disease.[5]

The needs assessment before implantation of this project revealed that DSME was not sufficiently provided, and the current diabetes education flow sheet was not used by care providers. The Institute for Healthcare Improvement MFI method was the QI design used for this project.[13,14] The MFI design has been used to accelerate process improvement work by numerous health care organizations successfully.[13,14]

The run chart used for this project manager graphically displayed data plotted over time and yielded data to make conclusions and detect process improvement. Overall, the run chart showed a nonrandom pattern/signal of change postintervention and after 2 PDSA cycles. The outcomes of the process improvement measure were evaluated, and the data plotted on a run chart visibly displayed an increase in the documentation of the provision of DSME on the diabetes flow sheet. The IPCP achieved the project's aim for provider documentation to increase from 0% to 100% (10 per 10 charts).

REFERENCES

1. American Association of Diabetes Educators. AADE7 self-care behaviors 2010. Available at: https://www.diabeteseducator.org/patient-resources/aade7-self-care-behaviors. Accessed February 17, 2017.

2. Centers for Disease Control and Prevention. National diabetes statistics report: estimates of diabetes and its burden in the United States 2014. Available at: https://www.cdc.gov/diabetes/pubs/statsreport14/national-diabetes- report-web.pdf. Accessed February 17, 2017.

3. Powers MA, Bardsley J, Cypress M, et al. Diabetes self-management education and support in type 2 diabetes: a joint position statement of the American Diabetes Association, the American Association of Diabetes Educators, and the Academy of Nutrition and Dietetics. Diabetes Care 2015;38(7):1372–82.

4. Kulbok PA, Thatcher E, Park E, et al. Evolving public health nursing roles: focus on community participatory health promotion and prevention. Online J Issues Nurs 2012;17(2). https://doi.org/10.3912/OJIN.Vol17No02Man01.

5. Haas L, Maryniuk M, Beck J, et al. National standards for diabetes self-management education and support. Diabetes Care 2012;35(11):2393–401.

6. Burke SD, Sherr D, Lipman RD. Partnering with diabetes educators to improve patient outcomes. Diabetes Metab Syndr Obes 2014;7:45–53.

7. Funnell M,M, Brown T,L, Childs B,P, et al. National standards for diabetes self-management education. Diabetes Care 2011;34(1):S89–96.

8. Chism LA. The doctor of nursing practice: a guidebook for development and professional issues. 2nd edition. Burlington (MA): Jones & Bartlett; 2013.

9. Institute of Medicine. The future of nursing: leading change, advancing health 2010. Available at: https://www.nap.edu/read/12956/chapter/1. Accessed February 17, 2017.

10. Hill J, Nielsen M, Fox M. Understanding the social factors that contribute to diabetes: a means to informing health care and social policies for the chronically ill. Perm J 2013;17(2):67–72.
11. Braveman P, Ererter S, Williams D,R. The social determinants of health: coming of age. Annu Rev Public Health 2011;32:281–398.
12. Braveman P, Dekker M, Egerter S, et al. Housing and health 2011. Available at: https://www.rwjf.org/en/library/research/2011/05/housing-and-health.html. Accessed February 17, 2017.
13. Langley JG, Moen RD, Nolan KM, et al. The improvement guide: a practical approach to enhancing organizational performance. 2nd edition. San Francisco (CA): Jossey-Bass; 2009.
14. Institute for Healthcare Improvement. How to improve 2017. Available at: http://www.ihi.org/resources/Pages/HowtoImprove/default.aspx. Accessed February 17, 2017.
15. Kent D, Melkus GD, Stuart PW, et al. Reducing the risks of diabetes complications through diabetes self-management education and support. Popul Health Manag 2013;16(2):74–81.
16. Anhøj J, Olesen AV. Run charts revisited: a simulation study of run chart rules for detection of non-random variation in health care processes. PLoS One 2014; 9(11). https://doi.org/10.1371/journal.pone.0113825.
17. Perla R, Provost LP, Murray SK. The run chart: a simple analytical tool for learning from variation in healthcare processes. BMJ Qual Saf 2011;20(1):46–51.
18. Hsieh HF, Shannon SE. Three approaches to qualitative content analysis. Qual Health Res 2005;15(9):1277–88.
19. Gumbs JM. Relationship between diabetes self-management education and self-care behaviors among African American women with type 2 diabetes. J Cult Divers 2012;19(17):18–22.
20. Bastable BB. Nurse as educator: principles of teaching and learning for nursing practice. 4th edition. Burlington (MA): Jones and Bartlett Learning; 2014.
21. Melnyk BM, Finehold-Iverholt E. Evidence-based practice in nursing and healthcare. 2nd edition. Philadelphia: Lippincott; 2010.
22. Lipson D, Rich E, Libersky J, et al. Ensuring that patient-centered medical homes effectively serve patients with complex health needs. Rockville (MD): Agency for Healthcare Research and Quality; 2011. 11-0109. Available at: https://pcmh.ahrq.gov/page/ensuring-patient-centered-medical-homes-effectively-serve-patients-complex-health-needs. Accessed February 17, 2017.
23. Summary of state patient-centered medical Home laws. Atlanta (GA): Centers for Disease Control and Prevention; 2013. Available at: https://www.cdc.gov/dhdsp/pubs/docs/state_law_fs_medical_home_laws.pdf. Accessed February 17, 2017.
24. Centers for Disease Control and Prevention: National Diabetes Surveillance System. Ohio diabetes 2010 fact sheet 2010. Available at: http://www.cdc.gov/diabetes/statistics/index.htm. Accessed February 17, 2017.
25. Maloney M, Auffrey C. The social areas of Cincinnati: an analysis of social needs. 5th edition. Cincinnati (OH): Patterns for Five Census Decades; 2013. Available at: http://socialareasofcincinnati.org/files/FifthEdition/SASBook.pdf. Accessed February 21, 2017.

APPENDIX 1: INTERPROFESSIONAL COLLABORATIVE PRACTICE DIABETES SELF-MANAGEMENT EDUCATION SESSIONS CONTENT

Part 1—initial IPCP group education session

1. Introduction
   - Overview of DSME actions to be taken by patients with diabetes to gain skills and knowledge to manage their disease and related conditions successfully.
   - Process incorporates IPCP goals for DSME and flow sheet documentation, IPCP experiences. Process guided by evidence-based standards.
   - Diabetes is a lifelong disease and requires self-management.
   - Diabetes is a lifelong disease and requires self-management.
   - Engagement: provide DSME based on person's life, culture, and experiences.
   - Solicit questions and respond to questions.
     - Ask about living with diabetes.
     - What is the most concern to you about diabetes?
     - How is diabetes affecting your life?
     - What can we do to help you?
     - What is 1 thing you are doing or can do to manage your diabetes better?
     - Discuss goal setting.
     - Teach back what is learn.
2. Use of the AADE7 tool
3. How to use of the diabetes flow sheet and its importance

Part II—menu to draw on in follow-up education of individual IPCP members
1. Highlight the IPCP approach to diabetes care—teaching-learning process
2. Risk factors for developing diabetes-related complications
   - Foot complications
   - Kidney disease
   - High blood pressure
   - Stroke
3. Current guidelines for diabetes management
   a. Glucose control
   b. Blood pressure
   c. Lipid management
   d. Dietary management

APPENDIX 2: AMERICAN ASSOCIATION OF DIABETES EDUCATORS 7 SELF-CARE BEHAVIORS

AADE7 self-care behaviors essential for successful and effective diabetes self-management are:
- Healthy eating
- Being active
- Monitoring blood sugar
- Taking medications
- Problem solving
- Healthy coping
- Reducing risks

Courtesy of American Association of Diabetes Educators, 2010.

Barriers to the Implementation of Pediatric Overweight and Obesity Guidelines in a School-Based Health Center

Lydia J. Yeager, DNP, MSN, RN, CPNP-PC[a],*,
Sharon M. Karp, PhD, MSN, RN, CPNP-PC[b],
Treasa 'Susie' Leming-Lee, DNP, MSN, RN[c]

KEYWORDS

- Childhood overweight • Childhood obesity • Pediatric overweight • Pediatric obesity
- Clinical practice guidelines • Barriers to implementation • School-based health

KEY POINTS

- This article aims to identify the barriers to the implementation of the 2007 American Academy of Pediatrics' Recommendations for Treatment of Child and Adolescent Overweight and Obesity in a school-based primary care setting.
- This project applied a quality improvement design using the Plan, Do, Study, Act cycle. An electronic survey was administered to nurse practitioners and licensed practical nurses working in school-based health clinics in New York. The survey assessed perceived barriers to guideline implementation and knowledge of, attitudes toward, and adherence to these guidelines.
- There were gaps in guideline knowledge and discrepancies in assessment, counseling, and treatment practices.
- The most commonly cited primary care–based barriers were lack of patient compliance, family lifestyle, and the poor dietary practices and sedentary behaviors common in America. The most commonly cited school-based barriers were that children have little control over the groceries purchased and foods cooked at home and the lack of parent presence during appointments.

Disclosure Statement: The authors have no relevant financial relationships with any commercial companies that have a direct financial interest in subject matter or materials discussed in this article or with any companies making any competing products.
[a] School Based Health Program, Ryan Health, 110 W. 97th Street, New York, NY 10025, USA; [b] Vanderbilt University School of Nursing, 366 Frist Hall, 461 21st Avenue South, Nashville, TN 37240, USA; [c] Vanderbilt University School of Nursing, 461 21st Avenue South, 216 Godchaux Hall, Nashville, TN 37240, USA
* Corresponding author. 110 W. 97th Street, New York, NY 10025.
E-mail address: Lydia.Yeager@RyanHealth.Org

Nurs Clin N Am 54 (2019) 159–168
https://doi.org/10.1016/j.cnur.2018.10.003   **nursing.theclinics.com**
0029-6465/19/© 2018 Elsevier Inc. All rights reserved.

INTRODUCTION

Pediatric overweight and obesity have reached epidemic proportions in the United States. In fact, more than one-third of US children and adolescents are overweight or obese, defined as having a Body Mass Index (BMI) at or above the 85th percentile.[1] In 2007, the American Academy of Pediatrics (AAP) published clinical practice guidelines for the treatment of overweight and obesity in children and adolescents. These guidelines recommend using a stepwise approach to the treatment of pediatric overweight and obesity, including prevention, such as healthy lifestyle choices; controlled weight management; all-inclusive management using providers from multiple disciplines; and tertiary management. The appropriate level of intervention, that is, step, is determined based on a child's age and BMI percentile.[2]

Researchers have found the use of the AAP guidelines to be effective in the treatment of pediatric overweight and obesity. In a meta-analysis of 24 randomized trials, combined dietary and physical activity modifications, similar to those recommended in the AAP guideline steps, led to small to moderate improvements in BMI in obese children.[3] Furthermore, residential weight loss programs, recommended in the Tertiary Care Intervention step of the AAP guidelines, have resulted in decreases in BMI and fat mass.[4] In addition, researchers have found that children following the AAP screen time limitations and physical activity recommendations were less likely to be overweight than their peers not following these recommendations.[5]

Many health care providers are aware of the existence of the AAP guidelines. Despite this awareness and evidence to support their use, there are gaps between these guidelines and what providers are actually doing in practice. As early as 2006, a study revealed that approximately 73% of nurse practitioners (NPs) working in family or pediatric general practice settings were aware of recommendations to screen for overweight and obesity using BMI.[6] However, these practitioners were not regularly using pediatric BMI percentiles to screen for pediatric overweight and obesity. In fact, only 9 of 82 NPs surveyed always calculated a BMI for children at least once a year and only 5 NPs surveyed used changes in BMI percentiles to monitor for disproportionate weight gain.[6] In addition, more than 40% of NPs surveyed were not using any guidelines whatsoever to direct their screening for overweight or obesity.[6]

Other researchers have also studied this phenomenon. During a chart review of well-child visits of 255 children, providers correctly identified only 34% of overweight and obese patients and provided only 11% of overweight and 26% of obese patients with appropriate counseling.[7] These findings were echoed in a 2011 study, which surveyed 96 hospital-affiliated pediatric primary care providers. These researchers found that although 83% of providers did use BMI percentiles, less than 25% and 35% of providers used the correct BMI percentile cut offs for overweight and obesity, respectively.[8] Furthermore, another study determined that pediatric providers correctly identified only 5% and 28% of overweight and obese patients, respectively, in patient charts.[9] Not surprisingly, the use of electronic medical records versus paper charts seems to improve provider documentation of BMI for overweight and obese patients[10,11] and will likely be a valuable resource in the screening for and management of pediatric overweight and obesity.

Not only are providers underutilizing the AAP's guidelines, but it also seems that providers may be overestimating their utilization of these guidelines. Surveys of pediatric providers and chart reviews found that although 93% of providers reported calculating BMI, only 73% of charts had a documented BMI.[12] In addition, only 22% of overweight and 51% of obese children were correctly identified as such in the charts. Furthermore, in these surveys, physicians overestimated their discussion of physical activity, sugary beverage intake, and appropriate history taking.[12] The aforementioned studies highlight the need for much improvement with regard to pediatric overweight and obesity guideline utilization in the primary care setting. Research has long shown that clinical practice guidelines improve quality of care, patient outcomes, and the consistency of care provided.[13] Thus, the proper implementation of these guidelines may improve the care provided to, and the outcomes for, overweight and obese pediatric patients.

Several barriers to the implementation of the AAP guidelines have already been identified in the literature, such as lack of time, lack of training, lack of resources, and patient and provider sensitivity toward the subject of overweight and obesity,[14,15] which may prevent or discourage providers from screening for BMI and using these guidelines in primary care. This is echoed by a survey of school nurses, which found not only that BMI was infrequently being used to assess for obesity, but also that school nurses did not feel competent in providing students with appropriate counseling.[16] There may be several unidentified barriers unique to school-based health centers (SBHCs) that are hindering implementation of these pediatric overweight and obesity guidelines. Identifying barriers to the implementation of pediatric overweight and obesity clinical practice guidelines may lead to the development of strategies to better enable implementation, thus improving the quality of care provided to overweight and obese patients in SBHCs.

METHODS

This project applied a quality improvement design, using the Plan Do, Study, Act (PDSA) cycle as a methodological framework to improve the use of the AAP overweight and obesity guidelines for children and adolescents in SBHCs. Participants in this quality improvement project were school-based NPs and licensed practical nurses (LPNs) working for a community health network in Manhattan, New York. There were 6 SBHCs within the community health network at the time of this project; each clinic was staffed with one full-time NP and one full-time LPN. The first author (LY) was one of the SBHC NPs and was not a participant in the project. Consequently there were 5 NPs and 6 LPNs who participated in the project. Inclusion criteria were working as an NP or an LPN at an SBHC in Manhattan that was part of a particular community health network. NPs were required to have a master's degree or higher, and LPNs were required to have a high school diploma and certificate from an LPN school. In addition, all participants were required to speak English. Exclusion criteria included working at an SBHC that was not part of the particular community health network, working at the community health network separate from the school-based health team, and being a different type of health care provider or staff member besides an NP or an LPN. There were no restrictions on participant age, gender, racial or ethnic group, marital status, or socioeconomic status. Of note, however, is that all participants in the sample were women.

This project used a staff survey to assess the barriers to implementation of the AAP's 2007 recommendations for the treatment of overweight and obesity in SBHCs, knowledge of these guidelines, current practices and adherence to these guidelines, and attitudes toward these guidelines. Surveys from previous studies in the literature review served as a guiding framework for the barrier and attitude questions. In addition, possible barriers unique to school-based health clinics, such as parents not wanting their children to miss classes or parents not being present in the clinic, were also included in the survey. There were 2 separate surveys, 1 for NPs (71 items) and 1 for LPNs (56 items), which were appropriate for each profession's scope of practice. Participants received a full explanation of the project and its purpose. No compensation for completing the survey was provided. Participant confidentiality was maintained by using Survey Monkey, an online survey tool, to construct a survey that protected the identities of the participants by deidentifying the data. The first author (LY) distributed these surveys from Survey Monkey through the community health network's secure e-mail system. The Survey Monkey software program stored the data generated.

RESULTS
Barriers

Several barriers were identified through the surveys of NPs and LPNs. Barriers were separated into those found mainly in primary care and those unique to school-based health. The most commonly cited primary care–based barriers by both NPs and LPNs were lack of patient compliance (100%), family lifestyle such as sedentary behaviors and poor eating habits (100%), and the poor dietary practices (100%) and sedentary behaviors (100%) common in American culture. NPs also most frequently cited lack of patient motivation (100%), limited parent motivation and involvement in the treatment process (100%), and parent refusal to recognize their child's overweight or obese status (100%) as barriers. In addition, LPNs most frequently cited insufficient community resources to refer to (100%) as a barrier.

Of those barriers specifically related to school-based health, the most commonly cited barrier by both NPs and LPNs was the fact that children have little control over the groceries purchased and food cooked at home (100%). NPs also most commonly cited the lack of parent or guardian physical presence during an appointment (100%) as a barrier (**Fig. 1**). LPNs also frequently cited that children have difficulty paying attention to counseling provided in the SBHCs (83.34%) (**Fig. 2**).

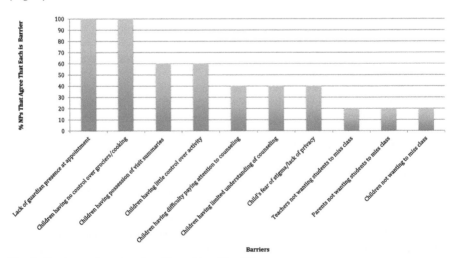

Fig. 1. Barriers unique to school-based health—NP.

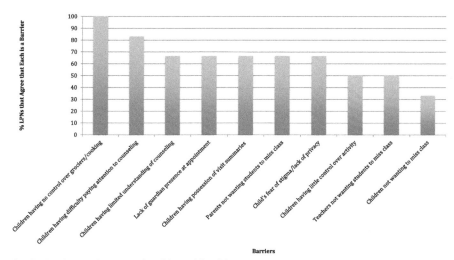

Fig. 2. Barriers unique to school-based health—LPN.

When asked about other possible barriers to guideline implementation in the school-based clinic setting, 2 NPs noted poor communication with primary care providers (PCPs) and having to direct patients to their PCP to obtain needed referrals. In addition, 2 NPs noted competing mental health issues and stress as barriers to addressing overweight and obesity. Another NP mentioned patient and family motivation and one LPN cited a lack of parent involvement.

When asked what would be helpful in the SBHCs to address these barriers, 2 NPs mentioned having clear, step-by-step protocols readily available in the clinics. Three NPs recommended additional services and resources in the school, such as mental health services, a nutritionist, and more staff. One NP mentioned finding ways to increase continuity between patients, parents, and the clinic. Two LPNs suggested more student and parent workshops to address this discontinuity issue and increase involvement of patients and families in physical activities and healthy lifestyles.

Attitudes

All LPNs and 4 of 5 NPs agreed that pediatric overweight and obesity is a significant problem in the United States, whereas 5 of 6 LPNs and all 5 NPs believed they could make an impact on the epidemic. All NPs and half of the LPNs were familiar with the AAP guidelines and believed that these recommendations could be effective in the management of pediatric overweight and obesity. Additional NP and LPN attitudes are included in **Tables 1** and **2**. Of particular note is that 4 of 5 NPs and only half of the LPNs believed they had adequate training to provide patients with proper dietary and physical activity recommendations and all NPs agreed that having practice recommendations and protocols readily available in the school-based health clinic would be helpful in their treatment of overweight and obese patients.

Current Practices

All NPs and 5 of 6 LPNs reported assessing and documenting BMI at least annually starting at age 2 years. With regard to health behaviors, all NPs reported assessing

Table 1
Nurse practitioner attitudes

Attitude	Strongly Disagree (N)	Disagree (N)	Agree (N)	Strongly Agree (N)
Measuring and documenting BMI is an important part of the assessment of pediatric overweight and obesity	0	0	3	2
I have adequate training to provide patients with proper dietary and physical activity counseling and treatment for overweight and obesity	0	1	2	2
I feel comfortable discussing pediatric overweight and obesity with my patients and their families	0	0	3	2
Having practice recommendations and protocols readily available in the school-based health clinic would be helpful in my treatment of pediatric overweight and obesity	0	0	3	2
I feel more comfortable treating other medical conditions, such as asthma and atopic dermatitis, than I do treating overweight and obesity	0	2	2	1

most of the recommended dietary and activity factors. Three of five NPs (60%) reported assessing frequency of eating outside of the home. Only 2 of 5 NPs (40%) reported assessing excessive portion sizes. All NPs reported counseling on most of the dietary and physical activity recommendations. However, only 2 of 5 NPs (40%) noted routinely counseling to remove televisions and other electronic screens from children's primary sleeping areas. Only one NP reported counseling on eating meals together as a family, allowing the child to self-regulate food intake, and avoiding overly restrictive feeding behaviors.

Table 2
Licensed practical nurse attitudes

Attitude	Strongly Disagree (N)	Disagree (N)	Agree (N)	Strongly Agree (N)
Measuring and documenting BMI is an important part of the assessment of pediatric overweight and obesity	0	0	4	2
I have adequate training to provide patients with proper dietary and physical activity counseling and treatment for overweight and obesity	0	3	3	0
I feel comfortable discussing pediatric overweight and obesity with my patients and their families	0	1	5	0
Having practice recommendations and protocols readily available in the school based health clinic would be helpful in my treatment of pediatric overweight and obesity	0	0	5	1
I feel comfortable weighing and measuring children	0	0	3	3

None of the NPs and half of the LPNs reported scheduling monthly follow-up visits as recommended when a child is identified as overweight or obese. In addition, only 3 of 5 NPs reported routinely ordering the recommended screening blood work for overweight children and only 2 of 5 NPs order the recommended blood work for obese children. There were also inconsistencies among NPs regarding when they chose to counsel parents to increase monitoring via logs of diet, physical activity, and sedentary behaviors; to refer patients to a comprehensive multidisciplinary team; to refer patients to a tertiary weight management center; and to counsel patients and parents regarding weight maintenance and/or weight loss.

Knowledge

All NPs and LPNs knew the correct age for beginning assessment of BMI. All NPs and 5 of 6 LPNs knew the correct BMI percentile for obese children. However, only 4 of 5 NPs (80%) knew the correct criteria for a normal BMI percentile, and only 3 of 5 NPs (60%) knew the correct criteria for an overweight BMI percentile. Only 2 LPNs (33%) knew the correct BMI percentile for normal weight and overweight children. In addition, only 3 of 5 NPs (60%) correctly identified the recommended screening blood work for an obese child.

All NPs knew when an overweight or obese child should progress from general dietary and exercise recommendations to increased monitoring. However, none knew that increased monitoring involves further reduction in screen time and referral to a dietician. Furthermore, none of the NPs knew that obese children typically have weekly visits when referred to a multidisciplinary team, and one NP did not know that tertiary care interventions should occur in pediatric weight management settings.

DISCUSSION

Evaluating the barriers to implementation of pediatric overweight and obesity guidelines will enable NPs and LPNs in SBHCs to overcome barriers unique to the school-based health setting. The surveys identified several issues within the SBHCs. The current practices of the school-based health staff do not align with the AAP guidelines. In addition, barriers identified in this project were similar to those identified in the literature. These barriers included those that school-based providers can control, such as provider and practice barriers, and those that school-based health nurses have little control over, such as patient and community or societal barriers.

Issues that can be immediately addressed are those that the school-based health providers can control, which are the provider and practice barriers. As the studies found in the literature,[14,17–20] some of the NPs and LPNs felt that they needed more training to provide patients with proper dietary and physical activity recommendations. These findings are also reflected in earlier surveys of school nurses, which found that school health staff did not feel competent in providing students with appropriate diet and activity counseling.[16] In addition, like the existing literature,[21] a major problem identified in the surveys was that the school-based NPs and LPNs do not fully understand the proper BMI percentile cut offs for normal, overweight, and obese children. Consequently, children may not be receiving treatment per the AAP guidelines simply because the providers do not recognize their overweight or obese status. Proper identification of overweight and obese students is vital to prevention and treatment. Furthermore, some of the NPs surveyed in this project reported that they do not know and are not ordering the recommended blood work for overweight and obese children. Consequently, continuing education focused on the management of overweight and obese children should be provided to the school-based staff. This training should include dietary and activity counseling and proper identification of overweight and obese BMI percentiles.

All NPs agreed that having a written practice protocol for the treatment of pediatric overweight and obesity would be helpful in the SBHCs. In addition, 2 NPs mentioned having clear practice protocols again when asked what would be helpful to overcome barriers to guideline implementation. Clear, straightforward protocols, including recommended blood work, should be embedded as treatment templates into the electronic health record system used by the SBHCs. This project found that, like previous studies,[14] lack of follow-up appointments was a significant barrier. Overweight and obese students were not being seen in the SBHCs regularly for follow-up appointments. Thus, regular follow-up appointments should be included as part of these treatment protocols. There were also large discrepancies amongst the NPs regarding when they chose to counsel patients and parents to increase monitoring via logs, to refer patients to comprehensive multidisciplinary teams, or to refer patients to tertiary weight management centers. These inconsistencies were also reflected in the assessment of guideline knowledge. Thus, the suggested stepwise treatments should also be assimilated into the treatment protocols.

This project identified barriers unique to school-based health that were not found in the literature, such as the lack of parent or guardian physical presence during an appointment and lack of communication with PCPs, resulting in poor continuity of care. Specific protocols encouraging increased communication with parents and PCPs during and after appointments and encouraging parents to accompany their children to the clinic if possible are ways in which these barriers can be overcome. These findings were presented to the school-based health team and obesity education sessions have been developed for the subsequent school year as a first step to overcome some of these barriers.

Interestingly, a lack of time identified by other researchers[6,14,17–21] was not one of the most frequently cited barriers. This makes sense; SBHCs have more flexible schedules because providers may call down students from class at times that are convenient for the clinic. Also unlike the literature, lack of health insurance[6,14] was not one of the most frequently cited barriers. This also makes sense, because SBHCs do not collect fees directly from patients or families, regardless of a patient's insurance status. These 2 factors emphasize the unique opportunities school-based health providers have to affect the struggle against the overweight and obesity epidemic in the United States.

Strengths and Limitations

Many of the reported barriers were similar to what is known in the literature. However, one of the strengths of this project is that it highlighted barriers that are possibly unique to school-based health. Another strength of this project was the length and detail of the surveys distributed, which resulted in a lot of information gleaned from respondents' answers. Furthermore, there were open-ended questions at the end of the survey, which allowed respondents to include additional information. However, a major limitation of this scholarly project was the small sample size and that project was performed exclusively at 6 SBHC branches of one community health network in Manhattan, NY, which limits the generalizability of these findings. Future quality improvement and research should seek to gather further knowledge of the barriers to implementation of the AAP's obesity guidelines in larger, more diversified samples.

Future Implications for Practice

The most commonly reported barriers were those largely out of the provider's control. In addition, this project uniquely highlighted the fact that children have little control over the groceries purchased and food cooked at home. Barriers embedded in cultural and home life contexts are more difficult to act on than barriers found within the clinics. However, possible ways to address these barriers, and future intervention phases for PDSA cycles, include sending home printed educational information regarding healthy eating, physical activity, and screen time with students after their appointments. In addition, as suggested by the LPNs, organizing student and parent workshops to increase involvement of patients and families in physical activities and to promote healthy lifestyles is a possible way to overcome these barriers.

Like a previous study, NPs also cited competing health care needs, such as stress and mental health issues,[21] taking priority over overweight and obesity counseling as a barrier. At the time of the survey, only 4 of the 6 SBHCs surveyed had part time access to social workers that address mental health needs. Some of the staff suggested increasing services, such as mental health services, as a potential means of overcoming this barrier. Although this is a costly and time-consuming solution, this may be explored in the future as a means of alleviating competing health care needs.

Another barrier uniquely cited in this project was the fact that children have difficulty paying attention to counseling provided in the school-based health clinics. The lack of parent or guardian presence in the clinic exacerbates this barrier, because adults are not physically present in the clinics with their children to hear and reinforce this counseling. This is further reflected by only 1 NP reporting counseling on eating meals together as a family, allowing the child to self-regulate food intake, and avoiding overly restrictive feeding behaviors. School-based health providers must be creative in addressing this barrier. Using motivational interviewing in the future may be an effective way to increase student engagement during appointments.

SUMMARY

Pediatric overweight and obesity is a grave public health issue in the United States. With overweight and obesity come significant physical health problems, psychological problems, social problems, and school problems. In 2007, the American Academy of Pediatrics published clinical practice guidelines for the treatment of overweight and obesity in children and adolescents. However, health care providers are not using these guidelines due to a variety of barriers already identified in the literature. Treatment of overweight and obese students in SBHCs presents unique problems; however, this has not been assessed in the existing literature. This project identified unique barriers to treatment in SBHCs, including lack of parent or guardian presence and difficulties in promoting continuity of care between the SBHCs and PCPs. From this work, we can begin to develop interventions to help address these issues within the school-based clinical setting. Identifying barriers to guideline implementation will empower school-based health providers to address these barriers, perhaps leading to the implementation of changes that transform these barriers into facilitators. These actions may improve the quality of care provided to overweight and obese pediatric patients, which could also lead to positive impacts on BMI and may improve health outcomes for overweight and obese children.

REFERENCES

1. Centers for Disease Control and Prevention. Childhood obesity facts 2015. Available at: http://www.cdc.gov/healthyschools/obesity/facts.htm. Accessed July 15, 2018.
2. Spear BA, Barlow SE, Ervin C, et al. Recommendations for treatment of child and adolescent overweight and obesity. Pediatrics 2007;120(s4):s254–88.

3. McGovern L, Johnson JN, Paulo R, et al. Treatment of pediatric obesity: a systematic review and meta-analysis of randomized trials. J Clin Endocrinol Metab 2008; 93(12):4600–5.

4. Gately PJ, Cooke CB, Barth JH, et al. Children's residential weight-loss programs can work: a prospective cohort study of short-term outcomes for overweight and obese children. Pediatrics 2005;116(1):73–7.

5. Laurson KR, Eisenmann JC, Welk GJ, et al. Combined influence of physical activity and screen time recommendations on childhood overweight. J Pediatr 2008;153(2):209–14.

6. Larsen L, Mandleco B, Williams M, et al. Childhood obesity: prevention practices of nurse practitioners. J Am Acad Nurse Pract 2006;18(2):70–9.

7. Reyes I. An evaluation of the identification and management of overweight and obesity in a pediatric clinic. J Pediatr Health Care 2015;29(5):e9–14.

8. Rausch JC, Perito ER, Hametz P. Obesity prevention, screening, and treatment practices of pediatric providers since the 2007 expert committee recommendations. Clin Pediatr 2011;50(5):434–41.

9. Dilley KJ, Martin LA, Sullivan C, et al. Identification of overweight status is associated with higher rates of screening for comorbidities of overweight in pediatric primary care practice. Pediatrics 2007;119(1):e148–55.

10. Bode DV, Roberts TA, Johnson C. Increased adolescent overweight and obesity documentation through a simple electronic medical record intervention. Mil Med 2013;178(1):115–8.

11. Keehbauch J, San Miguel G, Drapiza L, et al. Increased documentation and management of pediatric obesity following implementation of an EMR upgrade and education. Clin Pediatr 2012;51(1):31–8.

12. Chelvakumar G, Levin L, Polfuss M, et al. Perception and documentation of weight management practices in pediatric primary care. WMJ 2014;113(4):149–53.

13. Woolf AH, Grol R, Hutchinson A, et al. Potential benefits, limitations, and harms of clinical guidelines. BMJ 1999;318(7182):527–30.

14. Findholt NE, Davis MM, Michael YL. Perceived barriers, resources, and training needs of rural primary care providers relevant to the management of childhood obesity. J Rural Health 2013;29(s1):s17–24.

15. Walker O, Strong M, Atchinson R, et al. A qualitative study of primary care clinicians' views of treating childhood obesity. BMC Fam Pract 2007;8(1):50.

16. Nauta C, Byrne C, Wesley Y. School nurses and childhood obesity: an investigation of knowledge and practices among school nurses as they relate to childhood obesity. Issues Compr Pediatr Nurs 2009;32(1):16–30.

17. Jelalian E, Boergers J, Alday CS, et al. Survey of physician attitudes and practices related to pediatric obesity. Clin Pediatr 2003;42(3):235–45.

18. Klein JD, Sesselberg TS, Johnson MS, et al. Adoption of body mass index guidelines for screening and counseling in pediatric practice. Pediatrics 2010;125(2):265–72.

19. Small L, Anderson D, Sidora-Arcoleo K, et al. Pediatric nurse practitioners' assessment and management of pediatric overweight/obesity: result from 1999 and 2005 cohort surveys. J Pediatr Health Care 2009;23(4):231–41.

20. Story MT, Neumark-Stzainer DR, Sherwood NE, et al. Management of child and adolescent obesity: attitudes, barriers, skills, and training needs among health care professionals. Pediatrics 2002;110(s1):210–4.

21. Flower KB, Perrin EM, Viadro CL, et al. Using body mass index to identify overweight children: barriers and facilitators in primary care. Ambul Pediatr 2007; 7(1):38–44.

Printed and bound by CPI Group (UK) Ltd, Croydon, CR0 4YY

03/10/2024

01040408-0013